PHYSICIAN REVENUE SECRETS

CRUCIAL BUSINESS CONCEPTS FOR PHYSICIANS

MD EFFICACY
BOOK 2

MICHAEL MORKOS, MD

PRAISE FOR MICHAEL MORKOS, MD

Dr. Morkos is our most productive faculty member from a clinical standpoint (even while pursuing his master's program!), which I attribute to an incredible reservoir of energy and a complete mastery of the logistics of ambulatory care delivery, documentation, etc. Since joining our faculty, he has suggested multiple ways in which our processes can improve. He has a talent for seeing opportunities for process improvement and a real drive for continuous improvement. We have implemented some of his suggestions for efficiency, and our whole service line has benefitted. Dr. Morkos' clinical productivity is extraordinarily high, outperforming a full-time clinical target by 40%. A master of efficiency, he is always eager to contribute to projects that will improve patient care and/or clinic efficiency. He is highly sought after by his primary care colleagues.

— Melissa Cavaghan, MD, Service Line Leader,
Division of Endocrinology and Metabolism,
Indiana University School of Medicine

Dr. Morkos is extremely efficient in the clinic.

— Michael Econs, MD,
Chair of the Division of Endocrinology and Metabolism,
Indiana University School of Medicine

978-1-963244-05-2 Paperback
978-1-963244-06-9 Hardback
978-1-963244-07-6 Ebook
Published by MD Efficacy, Inc.

Website: www.MDEfficacy.com

Dedication

To Sandy, my wife, and Daniel and Anthony, my sons, who have shown me the beauty of family and its importance above any other achievements. You have brought balance to my life.

Mom, thanks for passing on your gifted math skills. It has helped me tremendously.

Dad, thanks for teaching me how to be detail-oriented and persistent.

INTRODUCTION

Many of us decided to pursue medicine for noble, often humanitarian, reasons. Perhaps you experienced the healing power of a physician or witnessed it on a loved one. It takes a considerable investment of time and money to reach independent practice, including many years of schooling, training, and, frequently, humongous loans. These values help ground and motivate us but banks, oblivious to the humanitarian values of medicine, need their loans paid back promptly.

In contrast, some choose medicine as a career because of its potentially high earnings. This view can also influence their choice of specialty or subspecialty.

As an academic endocrinologist, I get many rotating internal medicine residents in my clinic, and during inpatient service as part of their electives. Few of them, however, show an interest in endocrinology. Is endocrinology no longer attractive? I doubt it, the science of hormones is very intriguing. But, compared to other specialties, it does not pay well and my impression is that many are looking elsewhere for a higher-earning specialty to pursue.

For example, nephrology used to be a very competitive medical specialty years ago, not least as nephrology clinics would charge for every dialysate adjustment, boosting their revenue. When the Centers for Medicare and Medicaid Services (CMS) took over the payment for dialysis and decided to make it a "package payment", their income dropped significantly. Not coincidentally, many unfilled nephrology fellowship spots are now available yearly, even in the most prestigious programs.

So, it's clear that revenue plays a big role in career choices in medicine, even if it isn't often overtly discussed.

There are many emotions around thoughts and discussions of productivity and money, and I find them fascinating. Firstly, there is the guilt and shame in talking about money. It is as if physicians are expected to continue to work and provide the tremendous service they do, and not concern themselves with the details of their revenue, as they are relatively well paid anyway.

A second issue is a fear of insurance audits and the need to pay money back if overbilling is discovered. On the opposite side of the spectrum is greed, with some physicians working for extended hours and pursuing inflated billing to maximize their revenue. These issues raise questions around billing: What is fair? Do you fully understand the complexities of the billing process for the cases you manage? Can you defend your billing practices during an audit?

These questions are especially tough considering the billing and coding education provided to trainees is essentially none. Attending physicians can't be blamed, as no one has taught them even the basics of billing and audits. Shame, guilt, and fear also likely play a role. And, like DIY enthusiasts, they are left to learn by trial and error. When a simulated or actual audit happens, it is often a painful learning experience that results in a fear of future audits and a more conservative billing system.

This knowledge gap is in stark contrast to how we learn medicine. To build a strong building, you must first construct a strong foundation — the most costly and important but hidden part. This foundation takes time, effort, dedication, and investment to provide a basis for the structure it supports. Before we studied topics like internal medicine and surgery, for example, we needed to understand the first principles: physiology, biochemistry, anatomy, and pathology.

We certainly don't get anything like this for billing and coding!

During my fellowship, I heard of a two-day billing and coding course provided by an endocrinology society. I got excited, reserved a spot, and asked my co-fellows and attendings if they'd join me. As you might have guessed, no one was interested! Billing and coding were and remain a criminally overlooked area of expertise, and this course proved to be a valuable opportunity for me. I became the go-to coding expert for my attendings for the rest of my fellowship.

As physicians, our responsibilities are rooted in the investment in long years of study, self-development, and large loans. It is only right that we receive fair compensation. Considering increasingly expensive student loans and costs of living, a higher income is necessary to cover the bills. Without proper coding practices, physicians might either under-bill, leading to longer working hours and negative impacts on their personal lives, or overbill, risking severe consequences during audits.

What adds to the confusion are the big differences in

compensation models: the Revenue Value Unit (RVU) system, collections, bundled payments, and quality-based models in an insurance-driven system differ from the old straightforward fee-for-service model. Things are made even more complex by the levels of billing, various procedural Current Procedural Terminology® (CPT®) codes, and their requirements; as well as the different practice systems, including community-based institutions, academia, county hospitals, Veterans Affairs, and other private practice models.

Plenty of fuel for headaches!

When it comes to employment contracts, the compensation section is often not detailed, and a tempting sign-on bonus or initial guaranteed salary may initially attract applicants. However, complexities in compensation can lead to problems later, potentially provoking a costly job change that impacts many aspects of a physician's life. Conversely, physicians might overlook these issues due to an enticing offer. While revenue isn't the sole reason for job changes, it can be a significant factor for many.

I have a genuine passion for supporting and helping my colleagues get the most out of their jobs as physicians, a uniquely rewarding profession. On the other hand, it is heartbreaking to see overwhelmed physicians, working excessive hours to achieve their income goals.

In my previous 2024 book, *No Work After Hours*, I discussed various approaches to maximize efficiency and effectiveness during work hours to minimize out-of-hours work. In this book, I will explore various aspects of billing and coding, covering not only the technical details but also their broader impact on our work, lives, and careers as physicians.

Knowledge is power; just as you have mastered medicine, you must also master the business of medicine. No one will care as much about maximizing your revenue as you will!

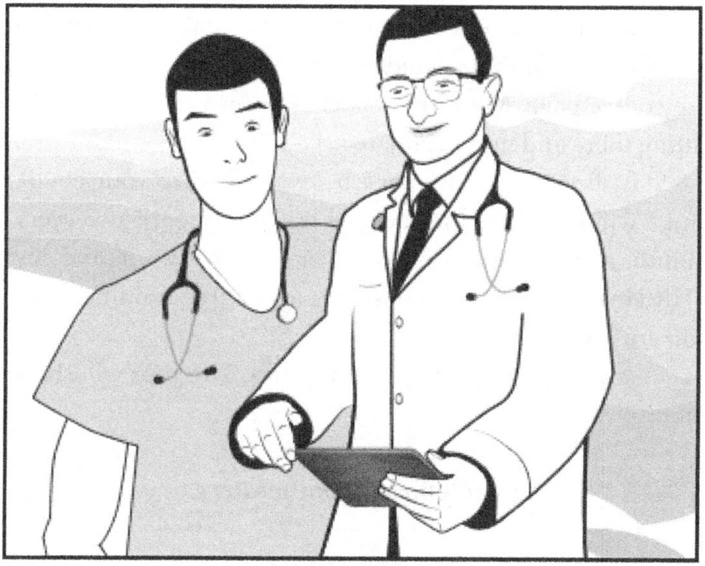

WHERE THIS BOOK FITS

This book is the foundation. It is the material I wish someone had handed me in fellowship: the terminology, the payment models, the compensation structures, and the logic behind billing an encounter correctly and defending it if you are ever asked to.

But a book has limits. It can explain medical decision making; it cannot walk you through twenty real encounters and show you where the level actually lands. It can tell you your compensation model matters; it cannot sit beside you and run your own numbers.

That is what I built the courses for. Physician Revenue &

Efficiency Mastery is the guided version of this material — the billing walk-throughs, the coding scenarios, the audit reasoning, and the efficiency systems that let me run the busiest clinic in my division without carrying work home.

It is CME-accredited, so your institutional allowance can usually cover it. Full accreditation and credit details are on the course page. Most physicians have unspent CME funds sitting there and never think to ask.

Start free. Go to the page below and leave your email, and I will send you the revenue tracking sheet I use every month, a short video showing you how to use it, and my EHR keyboard shortcuts. There is also a free training there you are welcome to watch.

Read the book. Track your numbers. The gaps will show themselves.

go.mdefficacy.com/mastery

Physician Revenue & Efficiency Mastery

1

PRACTICAL TIPS AND TRICKS

Money is 80% behavior and 20% head knowledge. It's what you do, not what you know.

— DAVE RAMSEY

Some physicians bill exclusively based on time, thinking it is the safest and least risky approach. Others charge 'moderate complexity' for everything, regardless of the complexity. They believe that being in the mean is safe. In contrast, others charge 'low complexity' for most encounters to play it safe but, as you will see in the examples below, this is not financially sound. Hence, I have dedicated an entire chapter (Chapter 7) to billing for outpatient and inpatient encounters.

In this chapter, I will focus on the financial aspects of billing to help you understand it thoroughly and make informed decisions by weighing it against other competing factors. I will start with some practical tips that you can immediately implement in your practice.

A lot of foundation needs to be built first, so I encourage

you to reread this chapter once you have read the whole book. It will make much more sense and consolidate your foundational knowledge.

Template Examples

Billing rules are similar in outpatient and inpatient settings. If you are still getting familiar with the work relative value unit (wRVU), I dedicated a section, Relative Value Units, to cover it in Chapter 4, **Business, Payment Models, and RVUs.**

Let us start with a clinic example and focus on how you can manage your template. The template is your design for the clinic flow, including established, new, and post-hospital patients, among other visit types and procedures. You get to determine the number of each per day, their duration, and distribution.

A good starting point is looking at how different patient scenarios can impact your schedule over an hour. We'll focus on regular outpatient encounters and provide a few procedural highlights, using the 2026 Centers for Medicare and Medicaid Services (CMS) wRVU rates.

Scenario 1:

- One moderate-complexity established patient (CPT® 99214; 1.92 wRVU) in 20 minutes.
- One moderate-complexity new patient (CPT® 99204; 2.6 wRVU) in 40 minutes.
- Total wRVU: 4.52

Scenario 2:

- Four low-complexity established patients (CPT® 99213; 1.3 wRVU each), each seen in 15 minutes.
- Total wRVU: 5.2

Scenario 3:

- Three moderate-complexity established patients (CPT® 99214; 1.92 wRVU each), each seen in 20 minutes.
- Total wRVU: 5.76

Scenario 4:

- One high-complexity established patient (CPT® 99215; 2.8 wRVU) in 20 minutes.
- Two moderate-complexity established patients (CPT® 99214; 1.92 wRVU each) in 20-minute slots.
- One additional procedure (e.g., continuous glucose monitoring interpretation CPT® 95251; 0.7 wRVU).
- Total wRVU: 7.34, *62.3% more than the first scenario.*

This breakdown illustrates how your total wRVU for an hour is affected by different combinations of patient types and procedures.

The Compound Effect

Small changes significantly add up in the long term via the **compound effect.** If your practice regularly operates like scenario four above, you will make much more revenue than practices adopting the other scenarios. Once you have mastered the billing guidelines, as detailed in Chapter 4, **Business, Payment Models, and RVUs**, it only takes a few seconds to determine the billing level and precise documentation phrasing.

It is important to understand the complexity of medical decision-making in billing does not necessarily match the duration of the patient encounter. For example, I commonly charge a high-complexity established patient (CPT® 99215; 2.8 wRVU) for short encounters, like 5-15 minutes, and a high-complexity new patient (CPT® 99205; 3.5 wRVU) for 15-25 minutes. I also often place an additional charge for a thyroid spectral Doppler ultrasound (CPT® 93880; 0.8 wRVU) or continuous glucose monitoring (CPT® 95251; 0.7 wRVU). These procedural codes are specialty-specific, and you need to master yours.

The two main ways to increase revenue are more assertive billing and higher patient volume. Ideally, you can do both, as they are not mutually exclusive, but it is best to focus on volume if you must choose one. To clarify this, let's look at a more extreme example from an endocrinologist's perspective.

If you see three established patients in an hour and charge high complexity for two (99215; 2.8 wRVU each) and moderate complexity for one (99214; 1.92 wRVU), you reap a total of 7.52 wRVU. On the other hand, if you add a moderate-complexity patient and charge the four as moderate complexity, this will come up to 7.68 wRVU, which is higher but has no high-complexity charges. Similarly, if you see four patients in an hour, with two moderate and two high-complexity, the total will be 9.44 wRVU.

This is why volume is a more effective revenue-increasing strategy than assertive billing, and if you *also* do the latter, this can significantly boost your revenue.

You might now be considering some stressful issues with these scenarios. For example, billing more higher-complexity charges will increase your risk of getting flagged and audited. Additionally, increasing patient volume might make you overwhelmed and burnt out with more out-of-hours work. All these issues can mean that your personal life pays the price of earning more money. Are there ways around this? What is the middle ground?

Firstly, as discussed in **Chapter 2: Emotions in Business in Medicine**, don't let fear hold you back. Instead, ask yourself: How can I optimize this for my practice?

As for the other concerns, I believe in efficacy, the combination of efficiency and effectiveness; you can see more patients, understand the correct complexity of your current patients (not that you have to see many more new complex patients) based on the current CMS guidelines, and finish everything on time. You can't, for example, suddenly jump from seeing 14 patients a day to 28 overnight. This won't happen, and it would not be a healthy pace of growth. But if you follow correct guidance and work on improving your workflow organically, it will happen slowly but surely.

Organic Growth

Remember years ago, when you were in middle school or high school, and you happened to look in a medical textbook? I remember it seeming so complicated. Then I heard a medical student brag about how much they were learning, and this made medicine seem even more unattainable. But, in due course, as I built my foundations, I was able to study and understand more and more complex concepts. Our foundation needs to be built slowly and carefully to raise and support a solid house. This applies equally to our medical practice and professional skills such as productivity. Learning to bill accurately is a single but important aspect of professional practice.

First comes clinical mastery; becoming a highly skilled physician who can achieve excellent outcomes. The next step is to master the skills needed to manage patient encounters effectively. Finally, focusing on increased productivity will be helpful once you have established the medical and social aspects of running a practice.

These skills are not mutually exclusive. We start learning them early in our career and they develop together. All these foundations can be lost if money is our main priority. For example, a patient who feels they didn't receive the appropriate therapy, has an unnecessary procedure, or experiences an avoidable adverse outcome or unpleasant clinical interaction, may choose not to return. Or even worse, they may publicly criticize you or get lawyers involved.

On the other hand, if a patient and some of their family members are your patients, as you are an excellent physician with great results and cheerful clinic visits, they won't mind a more expensive bill. They will also agree to see you for more frequent visits if needed.

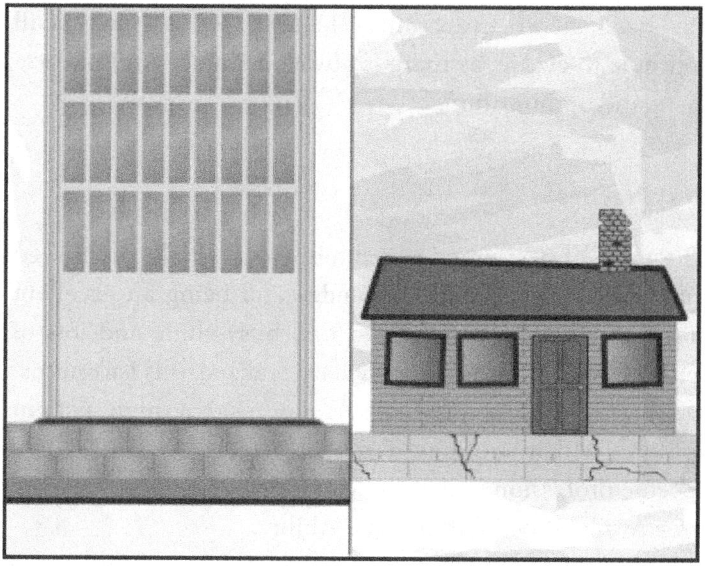

I still remember the first year after finishing my fellowship, when I spent a lot of time with every patient, trying to manage all their medical problems during the first visit! The patients were overwhelmed, and so was I. I would get even more frustrated when they failed to follow our agreed plans. As the years went by, I did this less and less and visits became shorter and more focused. This was a 'win-win' for the patients and me. They had less instructions to follow and I was able to see more patients and still maintain good patient satisfaction scores.

Again, developing such complex professional skills takes time to achieve an efficient yet balanced level of productivity. I'm not saying that it will take forever, and you can climb the steps relatively quickly as long as they are one after another and you aren't attempting to skip some. I'm biased, as I didn't have a mentor teaching me how to be productive, which might enable some 'shortcuts', so everything for me has been step-by-step. But I believe this is how I will continue to evolve, as there is always a chance for improvement and optimization.

Best Practice

The topic of best practice is interesting. Initially, I believed that mastering medical knowledge and being an excellent clinician would naturally lead to a busy clinic and lots of referrals. However, as you may have realized, this isn't necessarily true. To be productive, you need a high patient volume, which requires a robust referral system. Three specific professional qualities can help you achieve this: the 3 As: Availability, Affability, and Ability.

Availability: Be Available

Back to our hypothetical thyroid patient — imagine that the endocrinologist responded within a minute and told you what to do, but their first availability is in four months, and there is no way around it. How would you feel? Would you continue referring patients to them? Their practice is busy, and they may not be able to help you when you need them the most.

Availability is crucial.

When you start building your practice, you will have more time to communicate well and be available to accommodate urgent patients promptly. As time passes and your patient panel is full, it will get more challenging. Workflow tweaking ensures that you can accommodate urgent patients promptly, whether they are referrals or your patients with urgent issues.

One strategy I use is to freeze 20% of my slots for urgent issues in my practice so that half of them will open three weeks and the other a week beforehand. We have a well-run waitlist that will offer these slots to patients on the waitlist. This way, I ensure having a well-established system of running an available practice while continuing to be busy.

My practice is heavily focused on thyroid disorders, and like any endocrine practice, I have a big panel of patients with diabetes on insulin therapy. Many of these patients need close follow-ups, frequently in four to six weeks. The frozen slots give me this luxury, and I see them as planned. If you don't have a good plan and are booked six months in advance, you will do a lot of unpaid work between the visits, have more after-hours work, and hasten your burnout.

Affability: Be a Good Communicator

Having open communication channels and establishing good relationships with your colleagues and referral base is crucial. Consistency builds trust over time. This requires maintaining certain good habits, such as prioritizing electronic health record (EHR) messages by aiming to respond within minutes to a few hours, and at most within 24 hours.

Imagine that you are a primary care physician (PCP), and you see a patient in the clinic with a suspicious large thyroid mass noted incidentally on a chest CT. You want to refer this patient to endocrinology as soon as possible and send an EHR message to the endocrinologist. Surprisingly, they respond within an hour to take over the care of that thyroid mass. How would you feel about that endocrinologist? Pretty positive, right? They made your life easier and were a pleasure to communicate with.

On the other hand, imagine that they responded two weeks later, after the patient — who rightly wanted to be seen as soon as possible — had already found an outside endocrinologist.

I am not suggesting you have no work-life boundary and spend an inordinate amount of time trying to keep on top of communications. For example, I guide PCPs to use the EHR messages rather than pages as they are less disruptive. When not in the office, I use the out-of-office option, so they know when I'm unavailable. It gives the expectation that I will respond when I return, and they can use a backup referral for urgent issues.

Ability: Be a Competent Clinician

Let's imagine two different scenarios in our hypothetical case. After the endocrinologist saw the patient, they ordered a thyroid ultrasound and a biopsy that showed papillary thyroid cancer. The patient saw the recommended surgeon and had a total thyroidectomy.

Unfortunately, while preparing for radioactive iodine therapy, the pre-therapy scan revealed a 4 cm highly suspicious lymph node, and the patient necessitated a second surgery. The patient and her PCP were frustrated as the endocrinologist and surgeon could have easily picked it up if they had ordered a neck ultrasound preoperatively, which is the standard of care. The patient found another competent endocrinologist, and the PCP stopped referring patients to the initial endocrinologist.

Now let's imagine another scenario: the patient saw a competent endocrinologist who ordered a thyroid ultrasound and neck ultrasound for lymph node mapping at the same time, along with baseline labs, and got back to the patient right after these studies to review the results. They reviewed the images together, and the patient saw the suspicious thyroid nodule and ipsilateral lymph node. The patient understood the high risk of metastatic cancer, and the biopsy of the lymph node and suspicious nodule confirmed it. The surgery and radioactive iodine happened as planned, and the patient and the PCP were grateful for the endocrinologist's high-quality care, excellent communication, and availability.

The first two qualities we discussed above — communication and availability — are like the skills of a salesman. They can draw you in to buy the product, but the question is: will you return? It only depends on the product. If your clinical competency is robust, people will return, and others will hear about it. Alternatively, no one chooses to return to buy a poor-quality product, however good the sales pitch is.

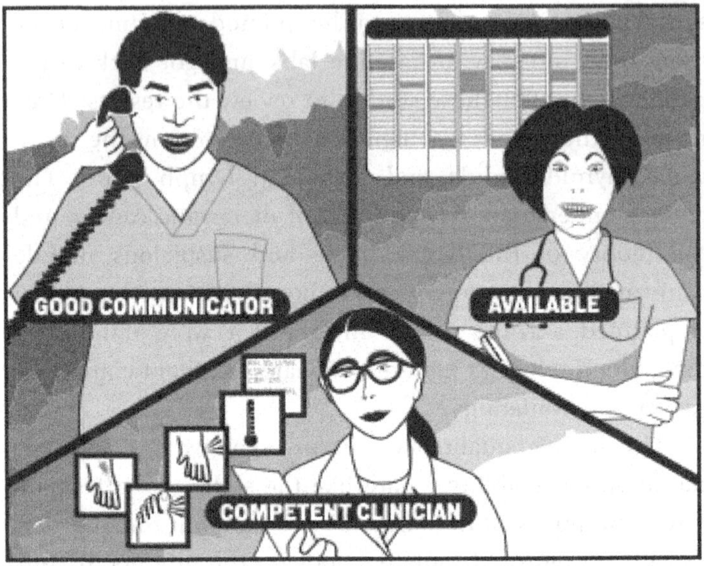

Practice Optimization

Our practice grows with us. Over time, it should improve as processes and updates are refined to meet our challenges. A stagnant practice is a declining one.

Understand Your Practice

The first step to improving anything is to understand where you are, i.e. situational awareness. How can you measure improvement without a baseline assessment? And why would you improve something without first knowing whether it needs improving?

Track Your Charges

To analyze and improve your practice productivity, you

need to keep track of what you are making. You don't want to be passively waiting for the report from your administrators or collections company to tell you how much money you have made. We are all human, and unintentional errors happen all the time. Also, no one cares about you and your income as much as you. I am not talking about advanced analysis; only simple steps are needed.

For example, I started with a simple Excel spreadsheet where I kept track of the patients I saw, one day at a time. The patients were named in the rows, while the top row showed the different charges with their wRVU values. If you go by charges, go by the *average rate of collections*. I made simple formulae to calculate my daily and cumulative revenue. As the months and years went by, I got data to track my trends and see the impact of the improvements I tried. This simple routine helped me refine improvements and get real results.

What started as a basic template evolved, and I came up with nice graphs, trends, and ways of identifying areas for improvement. Some basic statistics are also helpful to assess your situation, such as simple descriptive statistics like percentages, mean, and standard deviation. Just keep it simple.

The key to productivity routines is for them to become an automatic part of your daily clinical practice. Just like it is automatic that you have a panel every clinic day. You see them, place the needed orders, write your note, and place the charge(s). I recommend adding a simple step: write the charge in your billing spreadsheet, which will automatically calculate totals if set up correctly.

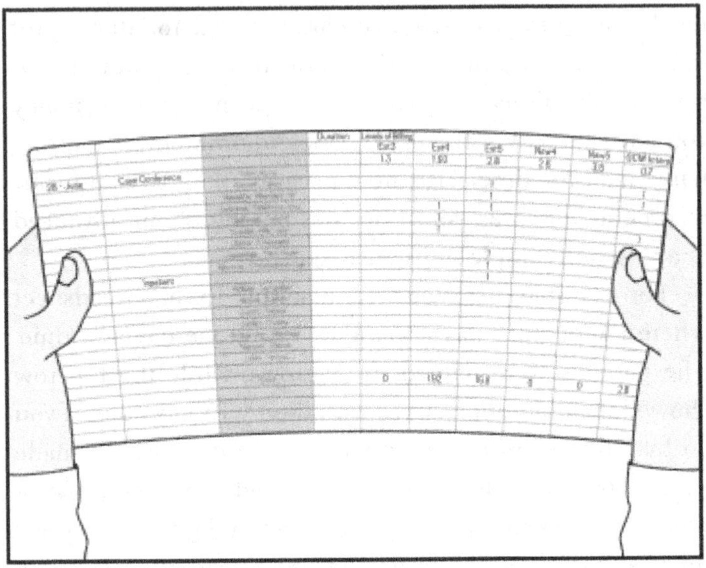

Besides helping you understand your practice, your billings spreadsheet will help you in discussions with your administrators. When you have a claim or complaint, you can now support it with your real-world data. For example, if you disagree with their revenue calculations, you can compare them with your data. Knowledge gives a lot of power!

Volume is Crucial

As we have discussed, seeing more patients is a crucial way to boost your revenue. The trick is to find the balance and not overwhelm yourself.

Many physicians feel overwhelmed when administrators pressure them to see more patients and maintain their benefits or revenue. Similarly, many physicians consider

EHR training overwhelming and begin to see clinical champions and clinical informatics teams as enemies.

I suggest consciously altering this point of view to see EHR and everything around it as an opportunity to improve clinical productivity. There are many advantages to EHRs that could never have happened during the old paper-based systems. (See my book, *No Work After Hours*, for more on improving efficiency.)

The next step is to increase your daily caseload one patient at a time. Add an extra patient slot and see if you can handle it. Wait until it feels natural, and then add another, etc. Similarly, I often make small iterations, then let things settle, to assess what works and what doesn't. If I feel overwhelmed, I revert to the last comfortable situation, stay there for a while, and then make another attempt in a new direction.

When the increase in volume is accompanied by mastering the art of understanding the right charges to place, your productivity will blossom. Do not feel you have to accept what is considered 'normal' or 'usual'. I had a colleague who told me that a certain revenue is 'the usual for endocrinologists in the US', and "no one earns more than that."

I didn't buy it and nor should you. As we have already shown, it is simple math that your revenue can be increased, but only if you invest in learning how and implement changes step-by-step.

Managing No-Shows

If patient volume is crucial, then 'no-shows' are a big problem. They also pose various challenges. If you try and anticipate 'no-shows' by overbooking, for example, this will help volume and revenue but if everyone shows up, your day will be challenging. As another strategy, if you challenge or 'fire' patients who do not show up, you will lose some of them. It is also uncomfortable for many of us to confront or 'punish' patients.

Hiring an administrator or receptionist to remind and confirm appointments is an expensive way of getting the job done. Labor is the costliest part of a practice, and it would be preferable that your staff's skills were focused on other work. Also, if you work for an institution, all you can do is make suggestions and hope that at least some of them are heard.

I have a few suggestions for managing appointment policy and no-shows:

Set Clear Policies:

- Arrival Times and No-Show Policy: Define strict arrival times with a reasonable grace period — e.g. 15 minutes for established patients and 25 minutes for new patients. Patients arriving late should be considered no-shows.
- Communicate Policies: Ensure that pre-visit notifications clearly state the **arrival time** and not the time of seeing the physician. This policy, like all policies, needs to be clearly communicated to all patients when they join the practice and at every appointment.
- Financial Penalties: If feasible, implement a financial penalty for no-shows to deter missed appointments. Even a small penalty holds value, although some institutions may opt against this approach.

- Dismiss Non-Compliant Patients: Consider dismissing patients with three no-shows within 24 months (for established patients) or two no-shows (for new patients). This helps manage liability and focus on patients committed to their care.

Manage Patient Expectations:

- No Exceptions: Front office staff should not make promises about policy exceptions. If a patient asks for leniency, staff should explain that the practice's policy is firm and avoid giving any false hope of exceptions.
- Automatic Notifications: Generate and send clear no-show policy letters after appointments, emphasizing the impact of missed visits on the practice, while demonstrating patient care.

Handle Exceptions Compassionately:

Give staff the authority to dismiss charges for legitimate reasons, such as emergencies or hospitalizations, and handle these cases compassionately.

Understand Patient Behavior:

Recognize that changing behavior is challenging and often driven by the pain of consequences. By setting clear expectations and enforcing consequences, you can encourage patients to take their health seriously. If patients do not commit, it may not be the right time for them to take their health seriously, and dismissing them can save you the liability of managing non-compliant patients.

In summary, effective management of appointment policies means setting clear expectations, enforcing consequences, handling exceptions with compassion, and being prepared to dismiss patients who do not adhere to these policies.

For example, I remember a 23-year-old patient with uncontrolled diabetes who canceled many visits and did not show up for two subsequent visits. When he finally did show up, I had a heart-to-heart discussion with him. I started by summarizing the facts, including that he has been getting care with me for two years, had had only three visits, and missed two recent visits. I then reminded him of the office policy of dismissal.

Lastly, I outlined his options; find another endocrinologist who can help him more than me, be dismissed if he misses a third appointment, or commit to his health and our policy, and I'd be glad to help him. Like what I saw with many similar patients, when pressured in this firm but compassionate way, he chose to commit to his health, didn't miss any further appointments, and his glucose control improved markedly.

Confrontations like this can be difficult but tremendously beneficial if handled well. I found the book *Crucial Conversations* by Joseph Grenny et al. very useful for learning how to handle confrontations by creating a safe environment and discussing facts and options sensitively.

Talking of psychology, I trust you are very familiar with the typical defense mechanisms people exhibit. Mature, responsible people tend to be fair and blame themselves for their mistakes. However, less mature people usually rationalize and blame others for their mistakes. The best way to help such people is to allow them to face the consequences of their actions. The danger as physicians is that emotionally immature people may well blame you for a complication of their disease or an adverse outcome while simultaneously not committing to your care. Hence, we need to be prudent and distance ourselves from such people. I would rather see patients with many comorbidities but who are more committed to their health and making their appointments.

A study I published in the *Journal of Racial and Ethnic Health Disparities* in 2021 on the factors associated with improved control of newly diagnosed type 2 diabetes showed that self-discipline, including commitment to follow-up visits, was crucial in achieving good outcomes.

You need to decide your professional threshold for defining a patient as a 'no-show'. For example, is it two hours before the visit, twenty-four hours, or twenty-four business hours? If a patient messages on a Sunday to cancel an appointment the next (Monday) morning, are they a no-show? The answer depends on how fast you can fill the empty slot. If your staff, for example, needs four days to fill an empty slot, set your no-show cut-off at four to five days.

On the other hand, if it takes six business hours to fill empty slots, then a 24-hour cut-off will work fine. Sometimes, the EHR reports can give you valuable data to assess this. Other times, you may need to collect and analyze your data to see the real situation. When I studied this in my division, the results were astonishing. It takes time and effort, but it is 100% worth it.

Automated reminders to patients are valuable tools. They can be via text messages, emails, or phone calls. You also need a user-friendly, customizable system for patients to choose their preferences as to how they are contacted.

Some companies are better than others at this, and I have experienced this first-hand. Regardless, automated reminders are well worth the investment and much cheaper than recruiting someone to call every patient to confirm their appointments.

Waitlists are another great tool for managing and filling the 'white space' of empty slots. As we discussed, availability is essential, and I recommend seeing patients at shorter intervals rather than doing a lot of extra work between visits. An **automated waitlist** can hold these patients in case of cancellations and automatically offer them available spots; a win-win for the patients and you. If you cannot afford an automated system, a manual waitlist managed by a dedicated administrator can also work. I say 'dedicated' as the job of everyone is the job of no one, and a single accountable person is far more effective than making it a shared role for a group of staff.

Overbooking is another option, especially for patients at high risk for no-shows. Your EHR can flag patients who did not confirm their appointments. Consider having an assistant call them or overbook these appointments. You may also consider overbooking patients with a history of prior no-shows but who haven't yet met the dismissal threshold. You can get innovative and try out different methods.

I recommend that you cap overbookings to the maximum number of patients you can see per session if everyone shows up. Refrain from overwhelming yourself, or you will be on a fast path to burnout! Also consider monitoring the data of your no-shows before and after every trial, like three months after, to assess if your strategy is working or if you need a better one.

If you like **virtual consultations**, as I do, and the payers cover them, consider using them to save some no-shows. For example, if a patient is already 10 minutes late for their arrival time, an assistant can call them to see if they are on their way. If they are not, offer a virtual visit and complete the rooming process during that short call. This way, you can still do the visit and save them a no-show. If it works well for you and your patients, it can become a routine policy.

Lastly, I suggest keeping track of your white space, no-shows, and last-minute cancellations. Scheduling appointments involves many technical details that we aren't taught, and the front office and checkout personnel tend to be the experts. If you are motivated, once you learn the basics, you can dig deeper into your data to improve your analysis. The more data you have, the better you will understand your practice situation and evaluate the effectiveness of your interventions.

I currently work for a large academic institution that manages thousands of physicians, and my strategies for improving policies for appointments and no-shows would take infeasibly long to implement. That's fine, I choose my battles, and I understand that their threshold for action is very different from mine. You will also need to understand your organizational limitations and what is possible in your situation. However, I can claim that my no-show rate is the lowest in my department and continues to improve.

In summary, here are the main strategies you can try to deal with no-shows:

- Adopt healthy boundaries.
- Enforce consequences for mistakes.
- Set reasonable expectations.

- Use "This is our office's policy" to clearly communicate policies.
- Dismiss established patients after three no-shows and new patients after two no-shows within 2 years.
- Send no-show letters and document them in the EHR.
- Establish a clear cut-off time for no-shows.
- Invest in a reliable appointment reminder system.
- Use a waitlist to fill gaps.
- Overbook with a manageable cap for high-risk patients.
- Offer virtual visits for potential no-shows.
- Monitor white space, no-shows, and last-minute cancellations.
- Choose your battles wisely.

Patient Portal Management

The patient portal can be an opportunity or a nightmare. I suggest cultivating it to be a harbor for your patients, where they can have a safe environment to share their concerns. Although it is legal to do so, I strongly advise you not to charge for these messages. It would give you only pennies but create a barrier preventing some patients from sharing legitimate concerns.

Ideally, have a nurse or experienced medical assistant triaging your portal inbox. Give them clear guidance on what should be considered automatically for a visit, what they can answer independently, and which messages to send you. Continue to educate them with every message, as this is how they will learn your system and become increasingly efficient. But from your standpoint, you need to give them consistent guidance to prevent them from getting confused and frustrated.

You also need a system that ensures you see patients sooner rather than later. If you ask the triaging nurse to avoid sending messages about urgent visits, ensure these appointments are arranged within a few days, not months. The same applies to lab tests. If a patient has an urgent test that requires attention and decision-making, you need to have a way of prioritizing them within a day or two. I prefer to finish everything during work hours to avoid after-hours work over the phone.

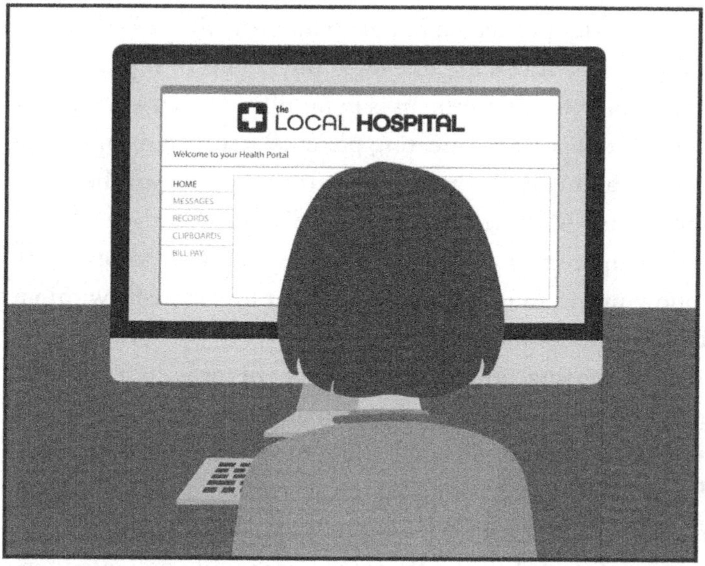

I always ask patients to do lab work and device data review a few days before their consultation. I set clear expectations that I only review results during appointments and not in between. If they are concerned, I'm glad to fit them into the schedule. This way, patients get excellent service as I talk to them during the visit, understand the circumstances behind the data, and make no assumptions.

On the other hand, this means I don't have to spend extra hours going through lots of data, necessitating patient phone calls, prescriptions, and follow-up lab orders. In my experience, patients are satisfied with this approach, as is evident in their satisfaction scores and their continuing to see me. I believe the core reason is that I set clear expectations compassionately.

See Patients Sooner Rather Than Later

It is important to accommodate patients within a few days to a few weeks. If you are like most physicians in the US, your next available appointment is in months or even a year. This delay is not good for meeting patients' needs and continuity of care and can also make for extra work for you between the visits. Although my practice is busy and the usual follow-up is in three to four months, I continue to see many follow-ups in four to six weeks and fit urgent visits within a few days, if not the same day.

My starting point for achieving this was to assess the maximum number of patients I could comfortably see per session, for example, 13. I then subtracted three patients from every session, making ten visits available for regular scheduling. Then I added these three slots back as '**frozen overbooks**', and the staff can only schedule patients there if I approve it. This became my template and provided a great cushion to accommodate urgent and timely visits and ensure reasonable availability. Two slots 'thaw' two weeks in advance and become available for the waitlist patients, and the third last slot thaws three days in advance to allow for patients I need to see back within a few days.

These overbooked slots also make up for no-shows and mitigate revenue loss without adding an extra strain. You can spread them out evenly across different time slots, to avoid having too many appointments scheduled back-to-back. This spacing helps prevent becoming overwhelmed and falling behind schedule. For example, scheduling overbooked appointments at different times within a single morning session (9 AM, 10 AM, and 11 AM) helps manage the flow of patients and reduces the risk of delays. It is a balance of revenue and timeliness.

I always strive to be, and generally am, on time. But some days are stacked with complicated patients, and I get behind, and I apologize to my patients. However, this should be the exception as our patients, like ourselves, have busy lives and their time needs to be equally respected. Being on time is a great way to do business, and we should all strive for this.

Patient Mix

You may need to consider a few aspects of the patient mix you are seeing.

Firstly, if you are compensated based on collections, the collected amount varies widely by the payers and your weight in the negotiation. For example, an institution with thousands of patients may have a stronger say in determining the reimbursement value than a solo private practitioner. That said, the latter should maintain their position in the negotiation.

Talking to private practitioners, it seems Medicare's payments represent the average rate. Some insurers pay more, some pay less, and a few pay far less. You need to pick your battles and choose the mix of patients you see. As mentioned above, patient volume is essential, but if the insurer barely breaks even, you should question whether it is worth the hassle.

Established patients usually generate higher revenue per time slot than new patients, especially if your time slots for new patients are double those for established patients. Additionally, the diagnoses often require different amounts of time per visit, and established visits may be made more efficient by using pre-visit templates and dot phrases (a predefined text snippet used in EHR systems). Also, as your career progresses, you may want to follow a niche interest and only see patients in this area. For example, I ended up shortening the duration of my new patient slots as I became more efficient, while also focusing on thyroid-related disorders. A balance is needed to accommodate new patients and maintain a relatively higher volume of established patients. As you develop, it will become more and more natural, and the volume of your established patients will grow. This is why physicians with longer years of practice earn more than fresh graduates, and this is a crucial point to consider when changing practices and starting from scratch.

Some patients may be more complex and less compliant with an insurer who barely pays the costs of the service. Deciding to decrease the volume of such patients in your practice or deciding not to see them at all is up to you. Some physicians have the calling, mission, values, and joy of serving these patients. Others may find it overwhelming as such patients may require significantly more time per visit, work in between visits, have a higher no-show rate, and have a lower rate of collections. A reasonable middle ground for many practices is to limit the number of such patients per clinic session, for example, a maximum of two. It is your choice if you have the luxury of making it.

Front Office

I hope you agree with me by now that being in clinical practice is indeed a business. An important part of running such a business is having satisfied customers. I am not suggesting that you become a people-pleaser — which is neither a realistic nor positive goal for physicians — but there are effective ways to foster a supportive culture that will better satisfy patients, even in challenging situations.

Front office personnel are key to setting the tone of the office and need to be warm, welcoming, smiling, and caring. A great and pleasant physician may get poor patient feedback simply because the front office personnel were grumpy and unwelcoming, either on the phone or in person. I have seen many instances of this.

Professionalism and warmth are both crucial for patient satisfaction. While professionalism can feel cold and impersonal, adding warmth and genuine care helps build a thriving practice that patients want to return to. They will often come with personal struggles or worries, such as facing a difficult diagnosis or struggling with co-pay, and a personal touch or brief but sincere conversation can have a large and lasting impact. Patients also appreciate opportunities for extra personal support, such as being able to leave a note for their healthcare provider.

Deductibles and co-pays are now the norm for many insurers. Most of us understand them well, but I will briefly explain it here for those who don't.

Healthcare insurers tend to pay large lump sums of money but want to prevent abuse; if something is 'free' there is a tendency to exploit it. To curb this, insurers have a **deductible** phase where patients cover costs up to a certain limit. Some services, like routine exams, may be free during this phase. Next is the shared responsibility phase, where insurers cover most costs (e.g., 80%) and patients pay a **co-pay**. Once patients reach their out-of-pocket maximum, insurers cover 100% of expenses, though some may cap this coverage. Coverage and thresholds can vary based on whether the doctor is in-network or out-of-network. Some insurers cover all costs up to a threshold, after which the patient pays until another limit, and then insurance resumes full coverage. This middle phase is sometimes called the 'donut hole'.

As you can see, it is quite a complicated system, and the coverage plans change often, like a moving target. Why is this important? Your front office needs to understand the various systems and each patient's situation and should collect payment, preferably before appointments. Some patients with high healthcare expenses will hit their out-of-pocket max early in the year, while others may be in the deductible phase for the whole year.

The current EHR systems come in handy here and can help tremendously. Many advanced systems have embedded revenue cycle management (RCM) software that can check the insurers' database in real time, pull the patients' plans, and decide their responsibilities. Be mindful that collecting co-pays is mandatory, and auditors will likely check for that. If you waive it, they may consider it insurance fraud. From an accounting standpoint, cash flow is crucial. The income may look great on paper, but it doesn't equate to actual money in the bank, and insurance companies can take up to 90 days to pay your bills. Generating bills is not free, so why not save money and time and ensure that the front office will collect the co-pays before the service? This cash flow is crucial, and you can significantly reduce the tedious work of chasing patients to pay their bills. Hence, I advise you to collect your money before appointments so you can pay your bills on time.

Give Feedback

Providing regular, consistent, and respectful feedback is crucial for a successful practice. You don't want to be someone who keeps things bottled up and then expresses them in passive-aggressive ways, eventually exploding after a triggering act. I used to be like this.

I used to notice problematic issues and mistakes, but I didn't want to hurt other peoples' feelings, i.e. I was a 'people-pleaser'. I would suppress my negative feelings, and they would pile up. I noticed instances of passive-aggression slip out, such as an unkind word or act, as if the suppressed frustration was spilling over.

Eventually, I would explode after a trivial act. In reality, it was not the act that caused me to explode, but the long-term accumulated frustration. The explosion presented in different ways, like firing someone, providing negative feedback to leadership, or having a nasty conversation. Usually, of course, others wouldn't understand *why* I was so mad. Eventually, I understood that I needed to mature.

The first step in providing effective feedback to staff is to have a clear vision of how you want your team to grow and improve. As a physician, you are the leader of your small team, and you need to keep your position as leader and not hand it to another person. Another aspect of this vision is that you need to care about the other person and want to help them improve. I became a better physician and person because of the feedback I received, although it was sometimes painful. Above all, I believe that patient care and maintaining a healthy work-life balance are crucial, and providing constructive feedback is essential to optimize both.

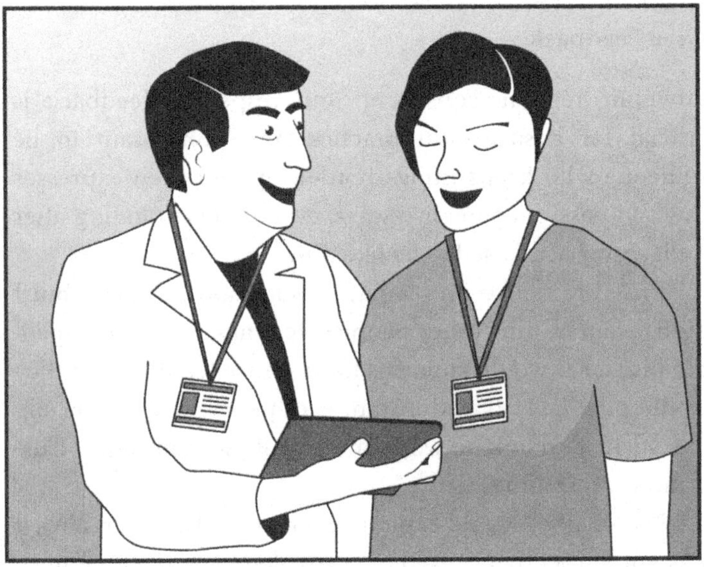

Effective feedback requires:

- **Foundations of strong relationships:** Effective feedback is easier with individuals you interact with regularly. For those you seldom see, involve their direct manager to facilitate communication.
- **Privacy:** Provide feedback in a one-on-one, private setting to ensure a safe and respectful environment.
- **Soliciting and Listening:** Ask for feedback on specific issues, listen to their perspective, and

then share your thoughts. This approach ensures they feel heard and helps address the issue directly.

- **Consistency**: Provide feedback consistently and follow up if problems recur. Escalate issues if necessary, but also recognize and praise successful responses.
- **Receptivity**: Be open to receiving feedback yourself; effective communication is a two-way street.

Mentorship

This topic is near and dear to my heart. Learning medicine is a process of discipleship and mentorship and we learn from experienced clinicians by absorption.

I regularly think of my mentors who taught me during rounds and discussions of patient cases and provided feedback on my notes. Mentorship is the shortest learning path, with fewer mistakes and greater potential than trial and error and reflecting on your successes and failures. We all make mistakes, those that don't are those not working!

In the modern era, there are other types of mentorships besides the classical route of an expert clinician and a trainee. We are in a great era of abundant resources, and the online world makes it far easier to seek and find knowledge. Artificial intelligence is another evolving resource. I found courses to be of special help, mainly because of the high-caliber expertise of the lecturers. I am still grateful for the billing course I attended during my fellowship, for example. It enlightened my path and helped me immensely with starting my practice.

However, courses or mentorships on physician productivity are rare. I don't recall, for example, discussing these topics during my training or as an attending physician. The only feedback one gets is from coders, through an internal audit, or in the annual coding updates, and they are often conservative.

So, how can I improve practice efficiency? How can I optimize my revenue? Am I charging correctly? Can I charge a higher level of complexity? How can I improve the clinic's efficiency? Should I go into academia or private practice? Will I earn more if I am a solo practitioner or a hired employee? How can I improve patient satisfaction scores while maintaining boundaries and sanity? How can I stop working after hours and maintain a good work-life balance?

Learning medicine is crucial, and it is the cornerstone of our practice. But these questions are also important, and I believe all training programs should educate trainees on these issues and the business of medicine. It would save a lot of physicians a lot of time lost to trial and error to understand important aspects of practicing medicine.

I have found it very satisfying when colleagues around me or those listening to my talks tell me that following my advice has significantly improved their practice's productivity, sometimes with remarkable results. Several started keeping track of their revenue and noticed areas for improvement. Others adjusted their templates to cut back on less rewarding patient types and procedures and saw subsequent improvement in their revenue. Most had a better understanding of the intricacies of billing and coding, and their coding practice and revenue improved.

We don't like big changes, and that's okay since they are often unhealthy. However, small changes, step-by-step can have a significant impact, which is why regular check-ins are valuable. I feel a personable approach is most effective, as everyone has unique backgrounds, goals, and priorities. I enjoy role modeling and learning from those who practice what they preach. Having delivered hundreds of talks, I understand that while speaking is straightforward, applying concepts in practice and maintaining an efficient, high-level practice is challenging. The true value of a talk comes from real-life experience, not just theoretical ideas

Teaching is crucial for learning and improving and combines a gift we are born with and a skill we must grow and refine. Some people are gifted in teaching, understanding the audience, attending to their specific needs, and having a passion for learning and well-being. Mentorship is most effective when it combines skilled teaching with a personal and caring connection.

Do you remember talking to a colleague who made you feel like a failure? Someone, for example, who kept bragging about their achievements and left you the impression that you could not become successful?

Humans are born ego-centric, and it takes years of maturing to get outside of this circle of ego. When focused solely on our success, we often strive to reach and maintain the top position. This is achieved in two main ways: being a high achiever or undermining others to elevate ourselves, and sometimes people do both. We should all strive to avoid this trap, as it is easy to fall into it. It is best to avoid both vain discussions and people who bring you down. It is not worth the time or effort. Instead, find mentors who practice what they preach, are high achievers, care about your success, and are gifted in teaching.

2

MONEY AND EMOTIONS IN MEDICINE

Fortune sides with him who dares.

— VIRGIL, *THE AENEID*

There are many mixed emotions around the business aspects of medicine for physicians. There are various reasons why the business of medicine is not taught in medical schools or training programs. One reason business education isn't included in medical training is the belief that, given the humanitarian nature of our work, we should prioritize patient care over financial concerns. Other reasons are that physicians don't want to appear greedy or consider it a private matter.

Unfortunately, this secrecy and reluctance to share productivity insights limits our learning and growth. Without sharing knowledge or brainstorming with others, we are left to our own devices to face these challenges alone. This also means that revenue payers can benefit from the lack of understanding, transparency, and oversight.

In school, many of us aimed to be at the top of our class by minimizing mistakes in our studies and exams. This mentality can persist after we leave school, leading us to strive for perfection in our clinical practice, continually fearing and wanting to avoid 'mistakes'. However, this approach does not apply to learning business. It is crucial in business to make mistakes, learn from them, and then make changes to improve performance. The more mistakes you make, the more you learn, and consequently, the higher your revenue. It is a learning curve.

How can we physicians face this fear of mistakes?

On the other hand, we have the ambitious among us who want to achieve the maximum possible revenue. They will charge the highest complexity whenever possible. I sometimes see the charges of other physicians and have been surprised by those charging for high complexity when their notes have poor documentation that won't support them. When they're audited, they will have a nasty surprise and may have to pay back a lot of money.

Being Rich

Many people who want to become physicians dream of being rich, driving a fancy car, and residing in a luxurious house. The overwhelming student loans might get in the way, but they still have this passion, which often influences their choice of specialty and subspecialty. When money becomes the master, it can easily ruin the life of its slave. We are not meant to be ruled by money but to use it wisely to enhance the ultimate good in our lives.

As an academic clinician, I meet many students and residents. Their first specialty choice is rarely a lower-paying specialty or subspecialty, and almost everyone aims to go to the higher-paying ones. It is rare to see medicine residents nowadays, for example, interested in endocrinology, rheumatology, or primary care practices. They are among the lowest-paid specialties. Instead, most are aiming for the competitive and high-paying ones. It has little to do with the appeal of a specialty's science and much more to do with revenue.

It therefore surprises me that whenever I ask a student or resident about billing and coding, I get very low-grade answers. This poor financial literacy extends from residents to attending clinicians. This needs to be improved.

Motivated by financial priorities, many trainees unfortunately choose high-paying specialties that do not fit their personality, gifts, or passions. They may earn more money but will live miserable lives. On the other hand, as is the focus of this book, clinicians in 'poorer specialties' can make far more money if they master the art of billing, coding, and adjusting their workflow to maximize revenue. Have you ever seen a primary care physician (PCP) earning more than a radiation oncologist without working before or after hours? I have.

Being rich is not wrong, per se. We have invested so much time, effort, and money into becoming doctors. What is wrong is to prioritize money and sacrifice what matters most. Each specialty is like a different culture with its own mindset and skills to attain and its passions to enjoy. Let me give a personal example.

I have a left-sided algorithmic brain that enjoys numbers. When I did the endocrinology rotation, I fell in love with it. The consistency of the hormonal feedback systems and logical adjustments strongly appealed to my cognitive style. When I did the infectious disease rotation, however, it was a whole other mindset. Instead of predictability and logic, it was a lot of imagination and gray zones about the wide array of differential diagnoses for every case. The infectious diseases specialists were so bright in a different way, but it certainly didn't come naturally to me.

My take-home point here is to master your business and make your professional choices based on your gifts and passions rather than financial concerns alone. You can make far more money while you're happy in what you do daily and living the lifestyle you chose, compared to being a rich, burnt-out physician who is doing everything to transition to an admin job as soon as possible because you are not in love with what you're doing. You deserve a better life!

Shame and Guilt

Although many physicians care about money, most don't like talking about it. Maybe because our job is so based on caregiving, discussing money comes with shame and guilt. While discussions in medical administration often center around financial issues, including reducing payments, at the front line it is shameful for us clinicians to discuss money. A rather pathetic situation!

Trainees fighting hard to go to high-paying specialties will rarely divulge that their main motivation is income. I love mentorship, and a part of my passion is guiding trainees to find their best fit. In some trainees, I sense that their underlying motivation is money, though this is often masked by the shame and guilt associated with discussing it. They are therefore surprised when I share details of what an endocrinologist can achieve financially, with the right know-how, as well as the surprisingly low revenue rates for procedures in higher-paying specialties. Their understanding also changes when I start discussing the lifestyle of each job and its requirements. At this point, they start to see the bigger picture.

This shame and guilt even extend to the leadership in medical education, who do not include the business of medicine in the curriculum. I run a rotation for our endocrine trainees entitled "Business in Medicine," where I share the various aspects of how to run a clinical practice, manage the workflow, and understand the intricacies of billing and coding. The rotating fellows' feedback has been very encouraging, and I strongly feel that this should be an important part of the clinical training for residents and fellows. How can you make an informed career decision when you don't understand the most important part of it: your pay?

Another aspect of the shame and guilt complex is how clinicians often take pride in the time they spend with patients to ensure thorough understanding, but they don't work on improving their workflow to be more efficient. As mentors, they also don't teach trainees how to work more efficiently, focusing instead only on being thorough. They do not emphasize productivity but instead encourage working after hours to ensure adequate patient care as if a physician's personal life is not as important as the patient's.

My point is that while a medical student might spend an entire hour with a single patient, an expert clinician can often address the issue in just a few minutes, highlighting the impact of efficiency and experience over time spent. The fixation on time rather than efficiency is a bad habit and a cultural problem that we are passing on to future generations of physicians.

I strongly believe in top-notch, highest-quality patient

care while maintaining good boundaries and not encroaching on my after-work hours.

Greed, Fear, or Fair?

Different emotions can accompany billing and coding. You can push for a higher billing level for every patient, as it will bring more revenue. From my perspective, greed is over-billing when a patient's clinical management and documentation doesn't qualify for that billing level.

Suppose your practice is focused on complicated patients who qualify for high-complexity coding and, therefore, the percentage is high. This is not greed; it is understanding your patients' complexity level. The key is to understand the complexity of your patients and how this matches billing and coding guidelines. Some complex patients need relatively longer visit times but won't qualify for a high-complexity diagnosis, while other relatively simpler patients will; you only need to understand the guidelines.

For example, a patient with cerebral palsy and a feeding tube who needs medication and feeding tube adjustments may only qualify for moderate complexity. Whereas a young patient with mild toxic multinodular goiter requiring a review of images and labs and who is starting methimazole (which needs intense monitoring for hepatotoxicity) will qualify as high-complexity. You can see that what we consider 'complex' may differ from the coding rules!

Fear is also common. Many of us are conservative in our approach and do our best to avoid the headaches and pains of audits. If your billing is more aggressive than the average for your specialty, unsurprisingly, you will be flagged and audited more frequently. Insurance companies are conservative and aim to minimize their spending. They constantly monitor for outliers and target those that will give them the greatest return.

How do audits work? Let's say, for example, that Medicaid is auditing your practice. You saw 2,000 of their patients over the past five years. They might review 20 patient records, and if they find that you overcharged in five of those records by $50 each, they could claim you overcharged 25% of their patients by $50 each. In this case, 25% of the 2,000 patients is 500 patients, so their calculation would be $25,000. You would then have to either repay this amount or enter 'battle mode', appeal the decision and contest the findings.

There is a good reason for this fear: the payback can be outrageous. Let us dive deeper into that. Remember when you were a medical student, and you saw a surgeon doing an extensive surgery with a high risk of complications? Or a physician intensely monitoring a lab result for a patient due to their severe disease? Did it fill you with fear when you imagined yourself in their shoes?

Knowledge is powerful; the more knowledgeable you are, the less fearful you will be. When you're confident, like you are now in your medicine and clinical skills, you can do great things with certainty. It doesn't mean no mistakes will happen, as we are all human, but they will be the exception rather than the rule.

Coders and auditors follow predetermined rules, and there are no surprises here. If your documentation reflects the level of billing, you are okay. The key here is whether you understand the billing guidelines well enough so that, before signing every note, you know what you are writing for the coder and auditor to defend your billing level. This may seem like a lot of work, but once you have this understanding, it only takes a few brief but crucial seconds and is often straightforward, as many phrases are standardized dot phrases.

Your attitude towards auditing can make all the difference in guiding your progress. If you see it as an opportunity to learn and improve your documentation skills and your revenue, you will continue to improve and try out new, more rewarding codes. If your reaction is to play it safe, you will become even more conservative and fearful.

Let me tell you a story: I was audited a few months after becoming an attending (independent) physician, and their language was aggressive. They directed me to pay back the calculated overcharges *immediately*. I was a novice, but the fighter in me was provoked. So, I reviewed all the patients they listed, and I prepared my argument. I responded with a carefully crafted and professional email, including clear evidence to support every charge they argued against. By the end of it, I paid nothing except a significant amount of time.

The lesson I learned from this experience was to simplify my language and use the *exact phrasing* as used the one used by the Centers for Medicare and Medicaid Services (CMS). As the months went by, it was clear that my billing levels were significantly higher than my colleagues, so my audits only continued. The next internal audit sent to me reported that I was 97% accurate, with one moderate-complexity patient 'mistakenly' classed as high-complexity.

As a perfectionist, of course, I wanted to double-check that everything was accurate. So, I reviewed this patient's case and, according to new regulations by the AMA that I had already implemented, I was correct. My score was updated to 100% accuracy. Since then, the auditing emails have been minimal, but I am pleased to see the annual coding lectures at my institution frequently contain snippets of my notes. My notes continue to get audited frequently, but everything runs smoothly. Isn't that great?

The concept of fair billing lies here: I know my services and the charge levels they deserve. I won't make things up just to overcharge; that is unethical. But I won't underbill either.

As we have discussed, the way to bill accurately and maximize your revenue is to use the language and phrases the auditors look for.

Celebrations

It is interesting to consider the things we as a profession celebrate and those we don't. In the academic world, the common awards are for the best teacher, the best researcher, and the best clinician. I have yet to see a 'Most Productive Clinician' or 'Best Workflow Improvement' award. It is, of course, important to encourage clinicians to teach, research, and improve their clinical skills. At the same time, we also need to encourage things that will improve a clinician's life.

Why is burnout so high among clinicians? Why do they work so many extra hours? Do they feel celebrated for providing outstanding, excellent patient care?

I know attendings who call patients to follow up on their routine lab results at 9 PM and another who will sign inpatient notes at 2 AM. How is their sleep quality? Are they fulfilled in their relationships? How do these faithful physicians handle their family lives? If they are married and have kids, are they satisfied with the time spent with their families? Are we celebrating the success of the physicians' families? Or is celebrating patient care far more important?

Let us take an example: a physician who makes $250,000 a year, works four full days per week, and otherwise has no face-to-face patient encounters. They have the luxury of three days off per week. Yet, the daily patient portal is loaded, averaging 40-50 messages and 20-40 lab results. They wake up early and stay late to see to these messages. This is the celebrated clinical faithfulness of promptly attending to their patients' needs. For a married physician, their family is suffering from their absence. The justification is that this is their calling and is how they earn a good salary and provide for their family. But, the physician's absence from their family can have a price that no amount of money can compensate for.

On the other hand, imagine a clinician at the same practice that has good boundaries and different priorities. They master their coding and billing well and make double the income for the same hours. They provide a significantly better income to take home. They know how to manage a practice better and celebrate patient outcomes without sacrificing their personal life. They can decrease the portal load to 10–15 patient messages per day, and most labs are done before the visits without additional follow-ups. They don't take any work home, so there is no work before or after hours. This clinician has prioritized success in the business of medicine, resulting in a far more productive, balanced, and happier life in and outside the clinic.

I suggest that if you find the values celebrated where you work don't align with your goals, create your own celebrations. I genuinely do not care about an award that will make me stray from my life goals and priorities. But if you set a great vision and celebration for yourself, you can become a lighthouse that leads others to a better life.

Seeing yourself thrive on your chosen path — increasing revenue and reducing after-hours work — is a rewarding experience. Spending quality time with loved ones and serving your community is invaluable. I deeply value the time I dedicate to my family and my church. These are top priorities for me, and I can only honor them if my work doesn't spill over into my personal time, allowing me to live out the values and celebrations that matter to me, rather than those dictated by others.

3

BASIC CODING TERMINOLOGY

The most valuable wealth of a man is his knowledge, which cannot be destroyed.

— THIRUVALLUVAR

To achieve good communication, you need a common language everyone understands. Humans understand spoken or written logical language using meaningful words. Computer language, on the other hand, is based on the zeros and ones of binary code. Computers can do so much based on these groups of codes; they can tell a story, ranging from diagnoses, ordered labs, and imaging studies, to charges.

My goal here is not to give highlights and convey the big picture of each type of medical code, along with some examples. The common ones you use will vary widely based on your specialty and practice.

ICD-10 Diagnosis Codes

It all started with the idea that we should speak a common language. For example, a physician may diagnose a patient with chest pain as a heart attack, another as angina, and a third will give a diagnosis of ischemic heart disease or acute myocardial infarction. All have the same idea but with different terminology and sometimes different details. Unifying the language, therefore, is useful. In addition, with the introduction of computer systems, databases care more about codes rather than descriptions.

This also helps insurance companies create rules for different diagnostic classes. For example, a certain medication can be automatically approved for type 2 diabetes but not type 1, or a certain procedure for certain diagnoses but not others. The list of reimbursement restrictions expands for hospital admissions, labs, and imaging studies. This is why selecting the right diagnosis is crucial, and it ultimately saves a lot of time and money.

The current healthcare system is very expensive, and health insurance companies strive to save money rather than agree to every expenditure. On the other hand, they would like to provide fair and reasonable coverage based on sound medical decisions. They therefore devised processes to filter the requests and strive to ensure that the expenditures match the preset criteria. Why should they, for example, pay for an off-label use of an expensive medication? Physicians may have their point of view, which can be reasonable and good from a trial standpoint, but systems don't work that way. The restrictions vary based on the insurance plan. More expensive plans generally offer greater leniency in approvals, while less expensive plans often have stricter criteria.

Another payment approach is bundled payments, which have been shown to be beneficial in saving money for insurers and helping institutions by ensuring a steady cash flow. (I elaborate further on this in **Alternative Payment Models** in Chapter 5.) For example, caring for a patient with only uncomplicated hypertension is different from caring for a patient with type 2 diabetes mellitus on insulin, with complications of retinopathy and nephropathy. The insurer participating in this model will give the healthcare institution a preset amount of money to care for each patient over an entire year, including all visits and healthcare needs. The different diagnostic codes are assigned different values, and the more valuable codes will earn more money. Imagine that the patient we discussed with type 2 diabetes was incorrectly assigned the diagnosis of Type 2 Diabetes Mellitus *without* complications. The institution would lose significant revenue, and the costs needed to care for such a patient would be much higher than the income.

Therefore, understanding the foundations of coding is very important. The International Classification of Diseases (ICD) system, which first originated in France in the 18th century to classify causes of death was later adopted by the International Statistical Institute, followed by the World Health Organization (WHO). Like every useful database, it grew vastly over the years with increased specificity and the ability to capture more details.

Let's dive a bit deeper into the ICD system and its details.

The ICD system is a tree-like structure, where each major category functions as the trunk of a tree, with subcategories representing its largest branches. These large branches continue to subdivide into progressively smaller branches until reaching the terminal smallest branches. For example, Circulatory System Diseases (I00–I99) serve as the trunk, Ischemic Heart Diseases (I20–I25) are a significant branch, and Acute Myocardial Infarction (I21) represents a smaller branch. If you use this code, more detail is needed, as there are decimal spaces for additional specificity. For example, I21.21 is for ST-Elevation Myocardial Infarction involving the Left Circumflex Coronary Artery, a specific diagnosis.

It is much better to choose specific diagnoses rather than less specific, big-branch diagnoses. This is helpful for everyone, including you. Our notes represent us and being precise and definitive is best practice. Your colleagues can see the high-quality care in your note; your well-chosen diagnoses can support your level of billing and specific codes are crucial for insurers paying bundled payments to capture the high complexity of applicable diagnoses. Many physicians have part of their revenue tied to them.

Luckily, most EHR systems will help you reach this level of precision.

If the diagnosis is unclear, it may be reasonable to initially code the symptoms, such as palpitations or weight loss. Our due diligence is to reach the diagnosis as soon as possible and update it accordingly.

We tend to use the same codes repeatedly. The initial effort is to choose the precise codes upfront and then use them repeatedly. Searching for or marking these diagnoses as favorites in the EHR is simple and fast and will become automatic as you continue practicing it regularly.

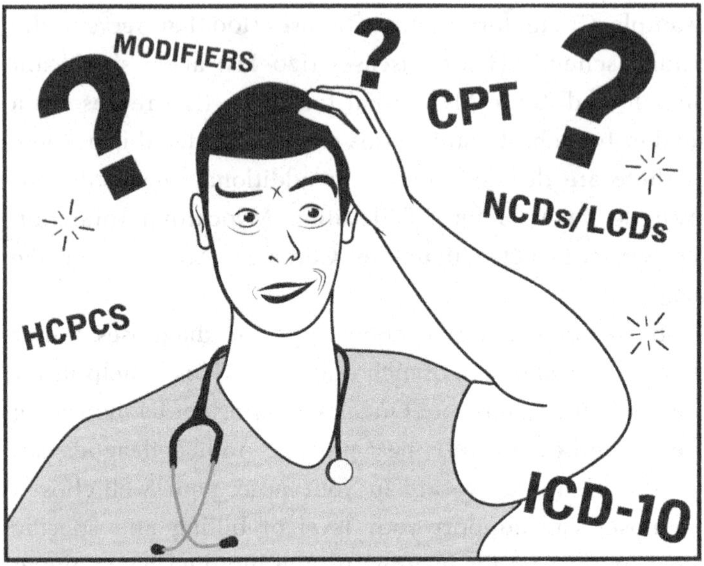

CPT® Codes

Current Procedural Terminology® (CPT®) codes are a huge and important codeset published and maintained by the American Medical Association (AMA). These codes are vital for billing charges related to physician-patient encounters, including inpatient and outpatient services, surgeries, anesthesia, pathology, and imaging studies.

CPT® codes complement the picture given by ICD-10 diagnosis codes, to make it clearer to insurance companies what is going on with each patient. For example, "the patient presented with [ICD-10 code] and we performed [procedure CPT® code]."

Each CPT® code is five characters long, either a number or alphanumeric. There are three broad categories, the most widely used of which is Category I, which encompasses the abovementioned areas. Category II is used for performance management, and Category III is a set of temporary codes for experimental technologies, services, and procedures.

Category 1 CPT® codes are divided into six sections, and I trust you can find where the ones you frequently use lie:

- Evaluation and Management: 99201–99499
- Anesthesia: 00100–01999; 99100–99140
- Surgery: 10021–69990
- Radiology: 70010–79999
- Pathology and Laboratory: 80047–89398
- Medicine: 90281–99199; 99500–99607

Each CPT® code has criteria and specifics you need to be familiar with. Sometimes, one code is better than another based on what you are doing. My suggestion is to master the codes you are using. **Evaluation and management (E/M) codes**, for example, are particularly used by outpatient clinicians. For new patients, codes 99203–99205 cover a range from low to high complexity, whereas established patients are similarly represented by 99213–99215.

Modifiers

Modifiers are two-character additions, letters or numbers, to add further detail. They append CPT® and Healthcare Common Procedure Coding System (HCPCS, see below) category-2 codes, providing additional information but keeping their description the same. For example, if I am charging for an additional minor procedure during an E/M visit, I must place modifier 25 on that E/M charge. Let's say I am seeing a new patient for thyrotoxicosis and performing a spectral Doppler ultrasound. I will charge 99204 (a moderate-complexity new patient) with modifier 25 and 93880 for the ultrasound.

Modifiers can provide additional details about a procedure, such as indicating laterality (e.g., RT for right and LT for left), specifying a body part (e.g., RC for right coronary artery and TA for toes), denoting an additional minor procedure performed simultaneously (e.g., modifier 25), or identifying a virtual visit (e.g., modifier GT), among other uses.

They are relatively simple but essential for accurate billing. You should pay close attention to them, as they convey important information and can occasionally affect your payment. Master the codes and modifiers you use most frequently and strive to minimize denied charges due to incorrect diagnoses, charges, or modifiers.

NCDs and LCDs

National Coverage Determinations (NCDs) and Local Coverage Determinations (LCDs) are decisions to grant, limit, or exclude coverage for specific items or services. Medicare determines NCDs nationally, while LCDs are determined locally by Medicare Administrative Contractors (MACs) in each jurisdiction.

These are important, for example, when you learn from your patient that the insurer did not cover a diagnosis of fatigue associated with tests ordered for vitamin D or testosterone levels, and they had to pay out-of-pocket. Many of them are logical, like an order for hemoglobin A1c (NCD 190.21) associated with a diagnosis of type 2 DM with hyperglycemia (E11.65), and will be approved.

I don't recommend looking up the NCDs and LCDs for everything you order, as this would be tedious and time-consuming. Instead, focus on these only when issues arise.

For services that are rejected or require additional refinement, review the relevant NCDs and LCDs to understand the covered ICD-10 diagnoses. Additionally, ensure that all ordered labs, imaging studies, and medications are properly associated with diagnoses.

HCPCS

You may also encounter HCPCS codes. They have two levels: Level I codes are the CPT® codes we have already discussed and are maintained by the AMA.

Level II codes, on the other hand, are maintained by the Centers for Medicare and Medicaid Services (CMS) and are primarily used to identify products, supplies, and services not included in the CPT® coding system, such as ambulance services, durable medical equipment, and many dental supplies.

4

BUSINESS, PAYMENT MODELS, AND RVUS

Formal education will make you a living; self-education will make you a fortune.

— JIM ROHN

Share of the Pie

The business of medicine involves many stakeholders, each pursuing their own interests and share of the pie.

Insurance companies will do their best to collect high premiums, negotiate lower payments for services, and increase bureaucracy with prior authorizations and denials to minimize their payments. They will also audit physicians and occasionally request a payback for inaccurate billing, doing their best to reduce payments. Healthcare systems will charge large bills to patients, especially the uninsured, and the facility fees are outrageous. The overhead cost of running such institutions is high, but they charge far beyond a reasonable profit margin.

On the other hand, patients may look for cheaper alternatives, and in-network providers minimize their out-of-pocket costs, sometimes at the expense of their health. Some may frankly ask their physicians for free services like lab checks and medication refills without visits. And, of course, we can't forget about the pharmaceutical industry charging outrageous prices for brand medications. Pharma are so good at business, for example, that they have been able to increase the price of insulin over the years — from $10 a vial in the 1970s to $300 in 2023 — *despite* the many generic forms available. I am impressed with such business acumen, but it is clear they frequently forget to consider the goals of reasonable and affordable patient care.

Amid this fight, where should physicians stand? Should we be the merciful angels who don't care about money, while working hard to satisfy everyone else?

Oh, yes, let's work ourselves into early graves to meet the targets set by our employers while filling out all the prior authorization paperwork and doing peer-to-peer talks to fight the insurance companies on our patients' behalf.... But aside from this battle, there is another struggle, where we continue to see pay cuts for physicians despite all the hard work, study and training we invested in getting to where we are today.

I don't believe that this is fair. We should aim to find a balance. We must strive, of course, to be excellent physicians, providing the highest quality patient care we can and maintaining excellent outcomes; this is our duty. At the same time, we need to recognize that medicine is also a business, and it should be as profitable as the substantial investment we made in our education and training. Our return on investment (ROI) should be very positive; otherwise, we're not getting our due.

Basic Foundation

The payment models in healthcare are multiple and complex. I will focus here on the US-based models, starting with the bigger picture:

- **Fee-For-Service:** This is the oldest approach. You pay for what you get. Some private practices will decline insurance coverage and accept cash-paying patients only. The physician payment here is straightforward so that income and expenses are clear.
- **Government-Based Payments:** This is represented in the Veterans Affairs (VA), where those who fought for the country are provided free lifelong healthcare coverage. The physician payment here is frequently based on a fixed salary.
- **National Health Service:** In this model, the government is responsible for covering the citizens' healthcare costs. The designed program is the Centers for Medicare and Medicaid Services (CMS). Medicare is federally funded, and Medicaid relies heavily on state funding, with partial support from the federal government. This model is comparable to Canada and England, where the government takes care of the population, except that it is not the sole model in the US.
- **Private Insurance:** Larger organizations are mandated by law in the US to provide insurance coverage for their employees. The bigger the organization, the better the deal. Yet, considering

the current outrageous healthcare costs in the US — which are by far the most expensive in the world — both the upfront costs (deductibles) and the maximum annual expenses patients may incur (out-of-pocket limits) are very high.

Quality-Based Payments

Insurance companies know their power and that the payer sets the rules. Whatever they say usually goes, and the wider their coverage, the more powerful they are. That is why the Centers for Medicare and Medicaid Services (CMS) drives most of the initiatives, and other insurance companies follow suit. Among other patient groups, for example, CMS covers all US seniors aged 65 years and up, so this is a *lot* of people.

Do you recall the Health Information Technology for Economic and Clinical Health (HITECH) Act that President Obama signed in 2009? It gave large lump sums, billions of dollars, to incentivize institutions to adopt the Electronic Health Records (EHR) system. It also had significant penalties for those who wouldn't. This achieved a great deal in modernizing the system and reminded the industry who really holds the power.

Payment models have also evolved over the years, from a simple fee-for-service approach, which encouraged delivering more services for higher revenue, to more complex models focused on enhancing quality and reducing overall costs. In these newer models, bonuses for high performers are funded by penalties imposed on those who do not meet the standards.

Bundled payments are another evolving trend that save insurance companies money. Institutions like them because they guarantee a consistent cash flow, and they can adjust their payment models and incentives to providers to maximize revenue. This includes payments for hospitalizations, surgeries, and annual patient care, among others.

Relative Value Units

In the early days, things were simple: name your price and charge it, and the patients who agreed to see you would pay, and that was it. As insurance companies continued to grow and expand their coverage, they needed standardization and a pre-set menu. This is how relative value units (RVUs) were developed, to ensure fair accounting for different services. RVUs provide a standardized way to measure services, with simpler procedures earning fewer units and more complex, high-risk procedures earning more.

There are three components of an RVU: physician work, practice expense, and malpractice components. Work RVU (wRVU) is the compensation for the clinical effort estimated for the corresponding billing level. For example, when writing this book in 2024, the wRVU for a level 4 established patient (99214), the most submitted charge for an established patient in an outpatient visit, is 1.92 wRVU. A level 5 established charge, 99215, denotes higher complexity, and therefore, its wRVU value is 2.6, 35.4% higher compensation than the level 4 established charge, 99214. The same concept applies to procedures: the more complex or demanding they are, the higher the reimbursement.

The wRVU values are publicly available via a page on the CMS website, which I suggest you bookmark to check regularly. As things change, it is good to check in with your coding department, get updates for the changes every year, and check this webpage as needed for your own specific, commonly placed charges.

RVU

((Work RVU x Work GPCI) + (PE RVU x PE GPCI) + (MP RVU x MP GPCI)) x CF

CF: Conversion Factor
GPCI: Geographic Practice Cost Index
MP: Malpractice
PE: Practice Expense
RVU: Relative Value Unit

The practice expense (PE) component of the RVU considers overhead costs, such as building rental and hired staff, among other fixed and variable expenses. The malpractice (MP) component is important due to the high liability expense of our work. Different services have different risks; therefore, this will be adjusted accordingly. The geographic practice cost index (GPCI) accounts for the different geographic locations in these three components, separately. For example, the overhead costs of a practice in New York differ from that in Indiana. Also, states may have different legislation that impacts the rate and cost of malpractice suits. One state may have favorable liability legislation but an expensive cost of practice, so it is important to keep them separate. The conversion factor (CF) is the amount assigned per RVU and determines the total reimbursement value, and CMS changes this often.

The wRVU-based system is a widely used payment model for physicians. It employs a standardized metric, wRVU, to assess productivity, providing a clear and consistent measure across the US. Even those using other models will also refer to the wRVU system. For employed physicians who are wRVU-based, there is frequently a set rate for the wRVU that will likely change over time. Private practitioners, on the other hand, focus on revenue collections and the payment rates from different insurers for various CPT® codes, which differ from the wRVU rates used for employed physicians.

For a typical private practice, the overhead can account for roughly 40–50% of revenue, and therefore, out of around $120 for a moderate-complexity established patient, the physician's revenue will be $60–$72. In comparison, the average wRVU rate for a reasonable institution can be $54 for a medical specialty. For the same level 4 moderate complexity, which translates into 1.92 wRVUs, this will come to $103.7, roughly a third more revenue.

Here, I will share my thoughts on this phenomenon. Some services bring a lot of revenue but need a solid referral base, e.g. radiology, lab services, infusion centers, radiation oncology, and surgeries. Medical institutions can earn significant revenue by establishing such comprehensive services. Physicians can't get direct revenue from them because this would be an anti-kickback statute violation. Therefore, the specialty-specific wRVU rate is set based on the specialty and the anticipated additional income from internal referrals and their utilization. Private practitioners can't get any side revenue from their ordered labs, imaging studies, or infusions unless they do them locally. There is a significant overhead cost for running them, and the volume assessment will justify whether it is worth the investment.

For the wRVU-based payment model, the calculation is usually simple. The physician will calculate the wRVUs they generated over the specified time interval and multiply it by the preset wRVU rate. It is that simple. What is complex but fascinating is to keep track of daily wRVUs, recognize trends, and see opportunities. For most physicians, it will suffice to get the monthly, quarterly, and/or annual reports, comparing them with the average. My advice is, "Don't be average!"

If you keep track of every charge you place, you will understand the monetary value and decide how to best use your time, while maintaining the best patient care.

Let me give you an example. I am an Endocrinologist, and I find bedside thyroid ultrasound exams valuable. The wRVU value for a thyroid ultrasound is, at time of writing, 0.56. It takes around 15–20 minutes to capture all the necessary images of the thyroid gland, including a minimum of 13 images of the gland itself and an additional five images for basic measurements and thyroid nodules. Writing the report and transferring the images takes another 5–10 minutes, adding up to a lot of time. In comparison, I can see two patients in 30 minutes with a basic charge of 1.92 wRVU each, frequently higher charging codes. What seals the deal is that my radiology department provides excellent images and reports, so I usually delegate thyroid ultrasounds to them.

On the other hand, I frequently do spectral Doppler thyroid ultrasound exams for new patients presenting with thyrotoxicosis. There is good evidence to support its clinical utility, and it takes me less than five minutes to do one exam and around two minutes to write the report and capture the images. The spectral Doppler thyroid ultrasound exams are unique, not formally done in regular radiology departments, provide valuable clinical information guiding management, and provide 0.8 wRVU each. It is a great source of productivity considering how quick it is to do and its clinical value.

You might think that 0.8 wRVU is insignificant, but once you start tracking your wRVUs, you'll be surprised by how the cumulative effect adds up. Small, routine changes have a significant cumulative effect in the long term. In this case, you might also ask: Thyroid ultrasounds are not cheap, so where is this money going? Or: Why do radiologists get paid so little for each?

These are sensible questions that deserve an explanation. There are two payment components for ultrasounds and similar exams: the technical and the wRVU. The technical component covers the cost of the machine and the revenue to cover the technician (not the radiologist) who performs the exam. The technician will capture images, label them, transfer them to the cloud, and draft a report. The radiologist will then review the images and the report, ensure they are correct, and then sign it. It can take them a couple of minutes, and they are done. This is why the wRVU is so small for a radiologist, as most of the money is for the machine and the technician.

Your calculation might be very different if you are in private practice and your income is based on collections. You don't need to concern yourself with all these components. You can do the thyroid ultrasound in 20 minutes and get paid $140, which may sound like reasonable compensation, so you will continue doing it. Additionally, having access to the ultrasound images can be valuable for clinical decision-making, especially when external radiologist images are difficult to access. By examining the clinical and financial aspects of various CPT® charges, you can optimize your workflow to enhance both productivity and efficiency in your practice.

I suggest you create a simple spreadsheet to track your charges. I started doing this a couple of years after starting independent practice. It has made and continues to make a huge impact. I recommend keeping it on a secure drive, preferably in your EHR system and include the patients' names and dates of service. This way, you can track your charges and investigate mismatches with your revenue cycle personnel. I also suggest doing it in real-time. Once I finish the note and place the charge, I mark my sheet with that charge. This minimizes errors, ensures no procrastination, and eventually becomes second nature.

One last tip: keep a close eye on your paychecks. Quality payments, payouts, bonuses, changes in effort, and other payments can go unnoticed. If you find something unexpected, reach out to your practice administrator or payroll to get some clarification. Also, ensure there is no discrepancy between what you expected and the actual deposits. No one else will care about this as much as you!

5

COMPENSATION MODELS IN PRIVATE PRACTICE

If you are going to be in business, you must learn about money: how it works, how it flows, and how to put it to work for you.

— IDOWU KOYENIKAN

How will your employer pay you? Will it be a simple or a complicated model? Can you calculate how much you will take home? Will it be fair? Which practice type is best for you? Do you understand the compensation section in the contract? Will you ask all the right financial questions during the interview?

And there are many other questions, of course!

This section aims to tackle the compensation part of various US-based systems. But first, I would like to step back and share a few thoughts. Money is important, but it is not the be-all and end-all. Why do you think burnout is so high among physicians? It was 38% in 2020 and increased to 63% by the end of 2021, according to a national survey co-authored by the American Medical Association. Of course, the COVID pandemic didn't help.

In a 2023 survey by the Medical Group Management Association (MGMA), the average length of time that new physicians stay in their first positions after completing their residency or fellowship is around two years, which is alarming. In this survey, the most important factor these graduates looked for was compensation, but this is not usually *why* they left.

Aside from the COVID-related challenges, I believe the high burnout rates and poor job retention are often due to people putting first things last and last things first, i.e. their priorities are upside down. I could write an entire book on this, but in essence, while income is important, it should *never* be the top priority.

We each have different gifts and passions, and when we apply them effectively, we are more likely to lead a fulfilling and innovative life. If we put money first, our professional decisions will be biased, and we may end up in a job or environment where we feel unhappy in our daily work. Prioritizing money in our decisions can also mean we lose the warmth and joy we initially experienced in a specialty we love, turning our practice cold. This is a sad story, and I truly hope you enjoy what you do and find satisfaction in your impact on your patients.

Okay, let's get back to business.

Collections-Based Model

The collections-based model is the most common model in small private practices. You see patients, submit the charges, and collect money from the insurance companies, the patients, or frequently, both. The collected amount from insurance companies will depend on your contractual agreement. In January of every year, the deductible phase starts, followed by the co-pays, and you need to collect money from your patients. Your ability to achieve efficient workflow and collect the money upfront from patients will decrease your chances of bad debts and lost revenue.

The way you calculate your take-home revenue is simple: income minus expenses. Your income is the money you collected from the charges you submitted. You need to do your best to maximize this part. Your expenses are also called 'overhead', which can be generally split into two components: fixed and variable. Fixed overheads are what you pay monthly, like a lease, utility bills, salaries, EHR costs, and equipment leases, etc.

Variable overheads are the expenses that will change from month to month. For example, inventory like probes for a certain procedure, and the amount used will depend on the rate of doing such procedures for that specific time interval. To run an efficient practice, you want to decrease overheads as much as possible. For a private endocrine practice, they are usually 35 to 50%. Salaries account for a significant portion of overhead, so it's crucial to balance hiring the right people with ensuring that you can afford them.

Clinicians can be innovative in navigating the overhead. The most expensive part is the clinical personnel. Outsourcing and using technology to automate processes may be cost-effective alternatives. Reciprocal scheduling is another option. For example, a practice with two surgeons decides that each surgeon will have two different days for the operating room (OR), when they won't be in the office. Surgeon A will be in the OR on Mondays and Tuesdays, while surgeon B will take Wednesdays and Thursdays. This way, there is no need to have a staff member for each surgeon in the clinic. The same can apply to medical specialties when virtual visits are feasible.

If you are an owner or partner in the practice, you can have significant tax advantages and write off some of your expenses. It can be rewarding, although you still have to pay a self-employment tax. Employed physicians pay the most in taxes, which comes as a package with the W-2 forms. On the other hand, payments based on work Relative Value Units (wRVUs) can be significantly higher than those based on collections for certain services, at least based on the pre-tax calculations, as I'll mention in the upcoming section.

wRVU-Based Model

The wRVU-based model is common for reimbursement in many private and academic institutions. Standardizing wRVU values for different CPT® codes by the AMA and the Centers for Medicare and Medicaid Services (CMS) makes it feasible and easy to implement. In addition, this means such institutions can use benchmarks to allow for competitive compensation in the market. There are several benchmarking tools, and academics tend to be more conservative than private institutions. The core of this model is encouraging productivity and rewarding the ability to see more patients and charge more, comparable to the fee-for-service model.

The next question is how much you will get for each wRVU, which is a difficult question that I will respond to with my personal opinion. There are ancillary services that can be a great source of income. These include labs, imaging studies, interventional radiology, infusion centers, and radiation oncology. When these services are offered in a hospital setting, the hospital can charge an additional facility fee that can be very expensive. A small private practice can't sustain paying $100,000 for a lab manager as the volume is too low. Point-of-care testing can add small revenue but not compared to the potential of a good lab. So, as a small practice, the main source of income is the collections. However, for a larger institution, the large volume justifies the overhead for these ancillary services.

The profit margin can be huge. A lab test may cost $0.50, but the patient may get a bill of $50. A Prolia subcutaneous injection at an infusion center, for example, may cost $3,000 to $9,000, based on the feedback I'm getting from my patients. A simple thyroid biopsy at a facility can result in a facility fee of $3,000 when the actual biopsy reimbursement for the physician is $69. A small practice won't get any of these profits. Similarly, when you refer a patient for surgery, the surgeon may get only $500 out of a $30,000 charge. There is an understandably expensive overhead for each of these services, but, still, the facility's profit margin can be very high if it maintains a high volume and well-run practice.

Ancillary profits may be why a specialty like hematology/oncology will get paid at a much higher wRVU rate than other specialties with a less lucrative need for ancillary services. For patients suffering from cancer, there will be many imaging studies, including PET scans and high utilization of infusion services, all bringing high revenue to the facility. Despite these services generating high revenue for the institution, the physicians receive only a small fraction of the total revenue, reflected in their higher wRVU rate.

Imagine a wRVU rate of $70, for example. For a level 4 established patient, 1.92 wRVU will result in $134.4, higher than the average Medicare rate for this level, $119.13. However, in private practice, this reimbursement from the payor ($119.13) is subject to overheads, which may take up about 50% of the total amount, drastically reducing the net income. Therefore, the institution is paying roughly $75 for every comparable visit. How can they afford this? By the millions of dollars that they make in collateral revenue.

As a private practitioner in a small practice, getting referral royalties from your neighboring lab facility or imaging center is illegal. Remember the anti-kickback statute? Giving gifts and percentages for referrals is legal in some businesses, but not in medicine. To get this benefit, you need to work for an institution, which comes with its advantages and disadvantages.

There is one pitfall here. Proceduralists can find it lucrative to have private practices and buy shares in their affiliated surgery centers. The wRVU value for many procedures is small compared to the total patient charge, which includes large facility fees. Buying these shares allows them to share in the profits from the facility fees. Without this practice model, they can't make any lucrative gains despite the relatively higher wRVU rate as an institutional employee compared to the collections without a share in the facility fees.

Salary

You may get a fixed salary or a pre-set hourly rate if you work for Veterans Affairs (VA), some county hospitals, other facilities, or in certain specialties. This model has its advantages and disadvantages. It guarantees that your income is stable whether the volume increases or decreases. It may be a great option for those who like stability and are risk-averse. On the other hand, it discourages productivity. Why would you see more patients when you can see less and get the same income? Why would you innovate and adjust your workflow to fit more patients in?

Many of these institutions will monitor wRVUs, collections, and productivity in the background. They may push underproductive physicians to see more patients. However, no rewards are given to those that are over-productive. It depends on your personality and preference. It is great that there are different models, and you pick what suits you best.

Alternative Payment Models

Given the changing paradigm in healthcare compensation models and the progressive shift to outcome and quality-based payments and bundled payments, compensation models will continue to change. This is different from the older fee-for-service model. In the old model, the more patients you saw and the more interventions you did, the higher the revenue. In the new model, the more patients you manage in your panel, the better target outcomes you achieve, and the fewer visits and admissions they have, the more money you can keep. I am talking from the institutions' standpoint, as they are the ones able to make these deals.

From the insurance company's perspective, the goal is to offer clients high-quality healthcare while keeping costs low. They use extensive claims data on diagnoses and related healthcare expenses to develop statistical models. These models estimate the medical complexity of patients and categorize various diagnoses into ranks known as Hierarchical Condition Category (HCC) codes. Patients with more valuable HCC codes receive higher reimbursements. On the other hand, patients with fewer comorbidities or fewer logged HCC codes, receive less.

The bundled payments system for institutions has several advantages. It is guaranteed and predictable cash flow, regardless of whether the patients show up for their visits. These institutions can implement procedures and incentives to capture as many HCC codes as possible to maximize their revenue from the bundled payments. They also have a large volume of patients to make up for the few patients who will need more services, resulting in higher costs, above the reimbursement value from bundled payments. They can also adjust incentive programs to attract physicians who will prioritize accurate HCC coding. Additionally, they may hire case managers to review patient charts and recommend any additional relevant codes.

From the practicing physicians' standpoint, it is a bit more complicated. If you think about a pure wRVU-based model, you can easily keep track of your wRVUs, multiply by the wRVU rate in dollars, and the calculated revenue is pretty accurate. On the other hand, these models are like a black box, and physicians can no longer calculate their revenue precisely. Physicians need to ensure they capture as many valuable HCC codes as possible. Doing so will affect their patient panel's risk score and, consequently, their revenue calculations.

Also, fewer in-person visits benefit institutions by lowering operational expenses and increasing efficiency, so they encourage remote management. This may work well if you compare your current volumes and reimbursement to the projected ones. You will do great if you modify your workflow to optimize revenue. The wRVU data will likely continue to be monitored in the background as an objective-established tool to assess productivity.

This model is like 'concierge medicine,' where patients pay a lump sum upfront and receive care as needed throughout the year. However, in this case, the revenue goes directly to the physician and their private practice, rather than to a larger institution. Additionally, while concierge medicine typically offers services from a single physician, this model may involve comprehensive coverage for various medical needs. It has the advantage of predictable cash flow, with the same benefits as bundled payments.

Quality Incentives

Quality incentives do not constitute a payment model per se but are a frequent component of compensation models. Considering the shift in payment models to quality-based and bundled payments, institutions are modifying their payment models to match this trend.

When payment is linked to certain metrics, physicians will do their best to fulfill these requirements to ensure adequate compensation, which is a positive for institutions. For example, insurers paying bundled payments rely on predetermined high-risk diagnoses to determine the payment amount. As mentioned earlier, these are called HCC ICD-10 diagnosis codes. Many institutions have incorporated the accurate recording of these codes into quality incentives for physicians to ensure they collect the maximum possible revenue.

Physician-to-physician, there are several disadvantages that I would like to share with you. The truth is that many employers, including CMS, aim for budget neutrality and don't want to pay you more. So, they ultimately cut back from your wRVU rate or salary to then give it back to you as a quality bonus, if you meet the requirements. This way, a portion of your revenue is based on an incentive to meet predetermined quality metrics. It's annoying, but that's how many people do it. Few institutions pay additional money on top of your pre-agreed- revenue as an incentive to achieve the agreed-upon quality metrics.

However, many quality metrics are reasonable, and we should strive to achieve them, regardless of such 'tricks'. In patients with diabetes, for example, we should start statins when indicated, ensure they get annual screening labs, and regularly check their feet. Vaccinations and screening tests should be done as well. All of these are reasonable.

Sometimes, unreasonable metrics are imposed, which is why having a well-chosen physician advocate is crucial to represent your group's interests. Generally, outcomes improve when achievements are accurately recognized and celebrated, through regular reports and incentives. However, when non-medical leaders enforce misleading metrics, it can lead to unnecessary frustration.

Compensation in Institutions

Institutions can vary widely from state to state and even city to city. There are general trends that I will share here, but my sincere advice is that you aim to have an in-depth understanding of the compensation model before you sign your contract. Similarly, once you start a position, stay up-to-date with the details of changes in the payment model, which always happen.

Earlier in this chapter, I highlighted some thoughts on small private practices under the collections-based model.

The next chapter will focus on compensation in academia, as it warrants a detailed discussion.

Firstly, many healthcare institutions in the US are classed as 'not-for-profit.' I would like to point out that this doesn't mean that they are not looking for profits; they most certainly are! They won't stay in business if they lose money, so they must look for profit to survive and thrive. What the term actually means is that profits won't be distributed to shareholders, but instead are invested in the institution's operations and growth.

Community-based institutions tend to be productivity-based, with incentives for achieving quality metrics. They are comparable to big private practices, and they celebrate good business, with regular reports featuring work Relative Value Units (wRVUs), revenue, and patient satisfaction scores. Research and teaching are not the cornerstones here.

County hospitals constitute a significant portion of the safety net for underserved and disadvantaged patients. They have a great mission to serve. In the old days, they were funded by states funded them and they were free at the point of care. Given rising healthcare costs, this model was unsustainable, and the waste was huge. The model shifted, and Medicaid provided coverage to documented disadvantaged patients. Many of these hospitals shifted to revenue-based compensation models for physicians or salaries with the wRVUs tracking in the background.

The nature of the served population of county hospitals presents unique challenges, including frequent language barriers, low health literacy, and difficulties with self-care due to social issues. Additionally, county hospitals have a distinctive organizational culture that aligns with the services they offer. Clinicians who thrive in these settings often have a profound passion for serving underserved communities. They find fulfillment in their work and are satisfied with the outcomes they achieve. However, this environment is certainly not for everyone.

The Veterans Affairs (VA) system is a unique governmental system where the government pays for the entire cost of healthcare services, and it has its own culture. VA hospitals have the benefit of not having to deal with insurance companies, prior authorizations, or peer-to-peer conversations. VA physicians tend to be salaried with a relatively lower workload than private community-based institutions. They usually work less and are also usually paid less. The leadership and hierarchy in the VA are comparable to those of other governmental institutions, and they are different from private institutions that thrive for increased business and profitability.

We are lucky in our profession to have different work models; physicians have many options. The task is to understand yourself well enough to find your best match, while minimizing biases, especially those related to compensation. You need to look at the whole picture and understand the organizational culture, including the unspoken policies. If you prepare well, you will end up happy in a position for the long-term.

Contracts

Contractual agreements are binding. Big institutions usually won't change their contract to accommodate your desires or wishes, but they may accept and make some reasonable adjustments. Your job is to understand all the details, ask about anything you do not understand, and do your best to negotiate. There is no such thing as perfection in life, but there are good fits. Like a marriage, there will be things you love and other things you (learn to) accept.

I hired a lawyer before signing my contract, but I found they did a far weaker job than I did in reviewing my contract, despite being highly recommended. Getting an expert's opinion is good, but you need to do your due diligence. In talking about compensation, the wording can frequently be vague and non-specific. In such cases, ask for written details, for example, in an email, that you can keep for future reference. Here are some questions to consider in analyzing your contract:

- What is the target wRVU for the proposed salary if it is productivity-based?
- What is the current dollar value of the wRVU?
- How often did it increase previously?
- What will you get if your productivity exceeds the guarantee in the first year or two?
- Can you get off the guarantee sooner, or will there be a penalty?

You also need to conduct a thorough market analysis to understand the average compensation for your specialty. This includes examining factors such as collections, wRVU rates, patient load, and work hours. Some details should be explicitly stated in your contract, while others may be variable and subject to change over time.

To gain a comprehensive understanding, consult with the practice administrator, physician leader, and practicing physicians about the various aspects of compensation. Perspectives can vary widely; for example, clinicians might praise the leadership or criticize frequent mistakes and model changes. Consider whether physicians typically earn more or less after moving beyond guaranteed compensation.

The more questions you ask, the more informed you will be. The goal is to have no surprises when you start the job!

Higher-Paying Specialties

Why do some specialties pay much more than others? Have you explored this and looked at the details of various revenues?

I find it very interesting. Let me share my opinion. Although patients and payers pay large lump sums for surgeries and procedures, they mostly go to the facility fees and ancillary services. A physicians' wRVU reimbursement for most procedures is not that much compared to large collections. What surprised me was that clinic visits, if done efficiently with appropriate coding practices, will yield higher revenue than surgical procedures. For example, a surgeon performing a total thyroidectomy will earn 15.0 wRVUs for a procedure that takes two to three hours. In an efficient medicine clinic, on the other hand, I can see six patients in two hours; for example, four moderate-complexity established patients (1.92 wRVU each), two high-complexity established (2.8 wRVU each), and perform a procedure (0.7 wRVU on average), giving a revenue of 14.0 wRVU. CMS adds to this a G2211 charge for most outpatient visits, which can be applied to these five patients, i.e. 0.33 each, making the total 15.6 wRVUs.

It was surprising to me that the wRVU value for surgeons and proceduralists is close to that for medical specialties within the same institution. But they tend to make more wRVUs, explaining their significantly higher income. How are they able to make that much when the surgeries don't add up to a very high wRVU value compared to clinic visits? For example, a full-time urologist can make 11,000 to 15,000 wRVUs, which is nearly double that of an endocrinologist's 5,000 to 7,000 wRVUs.

If an efficient medical clinic can earn that much, why do many endocrinologists and primary care physicians with low procedural loads make much less than surgical procedures? I have several thoughts about this. Surgeons and proceduralists tend to focus on the decision to intervene or not, and therefore, their visits tend to be faster and more focused. Proceduralists tend to be more decisive with relatively faster decision-making, resulting in faster encounters. Therefore, they can see a higher volume of patients per day. Culture also makes a difference: when a specialty is used to a certain income range, and billing changes happen with lower revenue, they adapt and adjust to maintain it. For example, surgeons used to earn a much higher income for surgeries, but as the revenue declined, they compensated by increasing the clinic patient load. Some see 30–80 patients per day to maintain their revenue. On the other hand, when clinic visits earn more, lower-paid medical specialties can see fewer patients and still achieve the same revenue. For these specialties, seeing 14 to 18 patients per day is often the expected average.

Medical specialties, aside from procedures, tend to require a higher cognitive load, more data processing, and frequently longer decision-making times. Additionally, clinic visits for medical diseases tend to be longer and chattier, and medical specialists are likely uncomfortable with shorter visits. Many of these physicians have hazier boundaries and tend to need help with patient calls, portal messages, labs, and work between visits. As you can see, I'm making some broad generalizations that may not always apply, but I believe these patterns are generally accurate.

I will conclude this section and chapter with the concept of **mindset**. With a progressive and curious mindset, you can easily be an outlier and achieve far greater success. On the other hand, if you 'go with the flow' and follow what everyone else does, you will receive average remuneration and find yourself joining others in complaining about the frequent pay cuts that we see every day. It is your choice.

6

COMPENSATION IN ACADEMIA

Not he who has much is rich, but he who gives much.

— ERICH FROMM

Medical academia is an interesting world with a wide variety of options for fulfilling different passions. My goal in this section is to provide a simple overview with a focus on productivity.

There are four main career paths in academic medicine: pure clinician, physician-scientist, physician-educator, and physician-leader. They are not mutually exclusive, and many academics do several of these. However, I quickly learned that the most effective approach is to focus on a specific path and develop expertise in that area; a jack of all trades is a master of none.

Regarding comparisons of remuneration, as we discussed in previous chapters, I suggest that you consider money as a part of a bigger package. Sometimes, for example, lower compensation comes with much higher job satisfaction, making the trade-off worthwhile.

The general trend in academic careers has shifted significantly over the years. In the old days, academics were salaried, productivity was unimportant, and teaching and research were the priority. The current trend is quite different, with business leaders in every department, and close monitoring of work Relative Value Units (wRVUs) and collections. Every academic clinician gets regular financial reports, with occasional meetings if there is inadequate productivity. It has become more like private practice, for many academic clinicians across different practice areas. Some institutions have kept the old model, but their salaries are far lower than average. Let us dive a bit deeper.

A full-time job is 40 hours per week, equal to 1.0 full-time equivalent (FTE). This is equivalent to five full days or ten four-hour half-day sessions. Therefore, a half-day session is equivalent to 0.1 FTE. Time in the clinic is called clinical fraction FTE (cFTE).

Other types of FTE include academic, research, and administrative. A physician-scientist will have a significant research FTE, a physician educator will have a dedicated academic/education FTE, and a physician executive will have an administrative FTE. It is important to keep a clinic, even if just a few hours a week, to ensure we don't lose our clinical skills. Even if we evolve in other endeavors, at the end of the day, we are physicians who treat patients.

Physician-Scientists

Physician-scientists are the ones leading clinical trials and big research studies. They have dedicated time to managing research demands, seeing patients as part of the trials' protocols, and writing grant proposals and manuscripts for publications. They also manage all the paperwork of clinical trials, oversee spending, and follow up with the institutional review board (IRB), a task that is getting more and more demanding. They also likely have a few weekly clinics to see their patients and possibly also do some occasional inpatient service.

Funding for research can come from public sources, such as the National Institutes of Health (NIH), or other smaller public organizations, or industry sources, such as pharmaceutical companies. The general trend is that getting grants is becoming more competitive, and funding is decreasing. If a researcher has a track record of successfully securing and managing grants, they are more likely to obtain future funding, which will constitute a significant portion of the physician's salary. If unable to get enough grants, physician-scientists may need to increase their clinics to make up for the deficit.

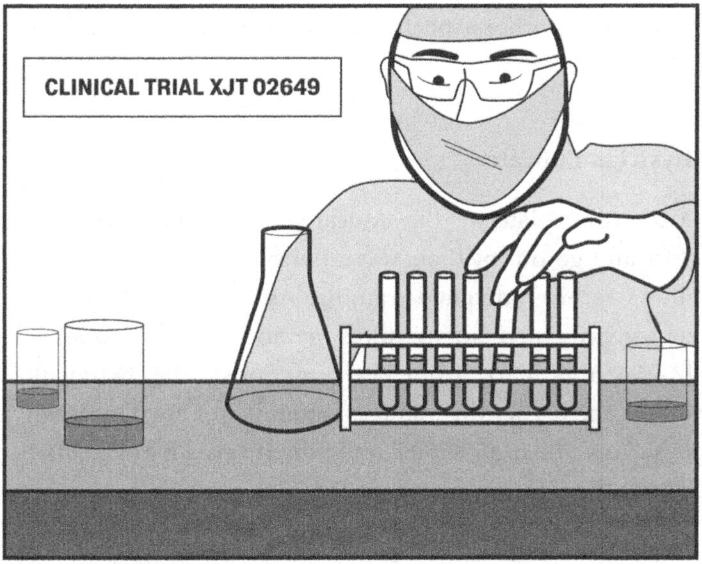

One appeal of the physician-scientist path is that it can come with a lot of fame if you are successful. They get to be recognized regionally, nationally, and internationally as subject-matter experts. At the time of writing, for example, talking at grand rounds can be rewarded with around $500 to $2,000 as honoraria. Physicians can also speak for pharmaceutical companies, but this is considered a conflict of interest and such income is capped at $25,000 per year in the US. Moreover, physicians who receive substantial compensation from pharmaceutical companies are generally prohibited from leading their own clinical trials. This restriction is in place to prevent potential biases or conflicts of interest and is a significant financial limitation.

Grants and honoraria usually result in less payment than a full-time clinician, frequently significantly less. The physician-scientist package has its advantages and disadvantages. I highlighted the financial part here, but I will discuss many other aspects in an upcoming career guidance book.

Physician Educators

I truly appreciate all the educators who spend time and effort and go out of their way to ensure that residents and fellows receive adequate training. As I have said before, I feel teaching medicine requires mentorship, where trainees observe and learn from their mentors. The better the mentor, the higher the mentees' training quality. This is why physicians are so precious, and why it takes many years to prepare them for independent practice.

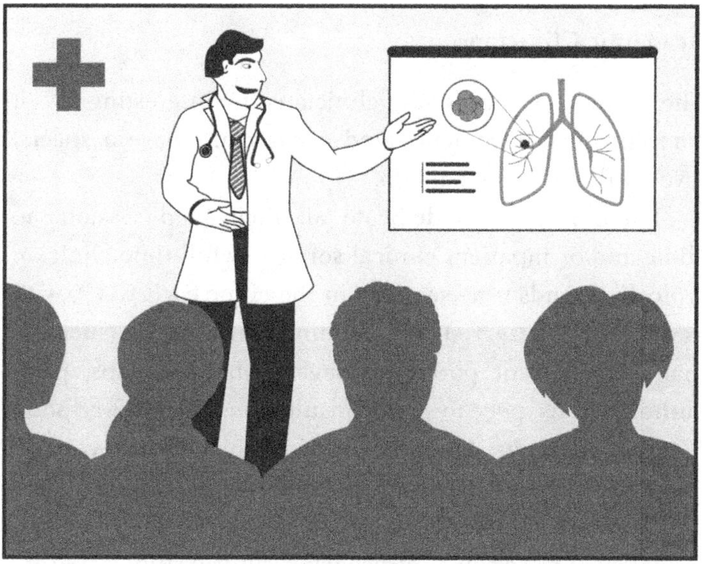

Teaching brings fulfillment, and those who are passionate about it find deep satisfaction in their daily work. Physician educators usually have some time paid to perform educational duties, including developing curricula, interviewing, leading educational sessions, and filing paperwork (and there is a lot of it!), among other educational tasks.

Typically, pay for educational work is significantly less than for clinical work, and the time needed to fulfill all the required tasks usually takes longer than the time paid. For example, after-hours time is needed to prepare for upcoming meetings or to write manuscripts in research studies related to educational endeavors.

Physician educators often find great satisfaction in their educational mission and may receive national or international recognition for their contributions. It can also allow for more time flexibility, for example, around family needs. It's a role with both positives and negatives.

Academic Clinicians

The model of academic clinicians is interesting as it combines private practice and academia. I have a special love for this as it is what I do.

These physicians dedicate all their paid sessions to clinic and/or inpatient clinical service. A full-time clinician typically spends nine sessions in the clinic each week, with one session reserved for administrative tasks such as managing patient portal messages, lab follow-ups, prior authorizations, peer-to-peer consultations, and prescription renewals. Despite being full-time clinicians, they often make significant contributions to research, teaching, and administrative duties.

Many of us conduct retrospective clinical studies. We are particularly suited to ask relevant clinical questions, as we see patients all day, every day, and a feasible way to answer these questions is by doing retrospective studies. Although they are usually not funded, they are relatively easy to do, have less complicated procedures, and are comparatively low-cost. Many trainees contribute, not least as the work will support their applications for future training. For the faculty, such projects add to their promotion dossier, which can provide some financial incentives, and can increase their national and international profile. This can open doors for possible industry-sponsored clinical trials, which may provide even greater financial incentives. Some academic clinicians opt for a diverse mix of activities to align with various interests, and these studies facilitate that balance.

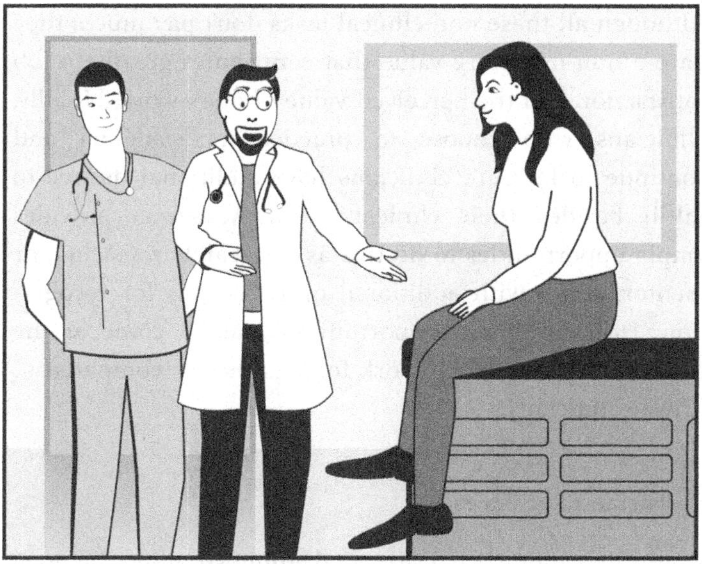

Academic clinicians also do a lot of clinical teaching, when medical students, residents, and even fellows rotate in their clinics or during inpatient care. Trainees in strong academic institutions are fortunate to learn from lots of different clinicians, each an expert in their field. Clinicians having expertise in a narrow niche usually have mastery of the ins and outs of their subspecialty. Tertiary care academic centers are privileged to have many such clinicians, and their trainees are fortunate to learn from the crème de la crème. Academic clinicians can also develop useful curricula, deliver lectures, and help moderate medical student teaching sessions. Many universities try to reward the teaching faculty by providing educational RVUs (eRVUs), though they typically have far less value than wRVUs.

Clinicians in academia can also help with administrative activities and in developing protocols in the clinic. As you can see, they have a pivotal role in academia.

Although all these non-clinical tasks don't pay much, they have a non-monetary value that contributes greatly to job satisfaction and the perceived value of one's work. Usually, clinicians who choose to practice in academia and continue to be pure clinicians have additional desires to fulfill besides their clinical work. Academia provides ample opportunities to do this as a researcher, teacher, or mentor, along with additional opportunities for recognition. However, these opportunities usually come at the expense of doing more work for less money compared to private clinicians.

Physician Executives

Every clinical practice needs good administration. The practice leader can make it or break it; a good leader can nourish a supportive and positive culture that makes the practice appealing to the physicians and other staff. And a bad leader can turn a pleasant practice into a nightmare.

You may have noticed, as I have, that many clinicians prefer to be led rather than to stand up and be leaders themselves. So, when the culture becomes toxic, the easiest option for many is to leave and look for another job. Few entrepreneurial clinicians enter academia, as most physicians with strong executive drive typically pursue private practice from the start of their careers.

Additionally, most current academic institutions use clinical money to support their academic mission. Believe it or not, some institutions impose formal deductions on academic clinicians, often taken from the wRVU value, to support their school of medicine's research and teaching missions. Other institutions start with a lower wRVU rate than the national average, creating another revenue stream to support the academic mission. This gives you an idea of why clinical work is important and has to be well-managed.

There are clinic managers, hired staff, monitored schedules, and wRVU reports to assess the various clinic utilizations and identify opportunities for improvement. The goal is to maximize revenue while providing adequate support with reasonable expenses. This is comparable to private institutions. What distinguishes academic centers is the number and level of expert sub-specialists who can care for complex patients needing intensive and costly therapies.

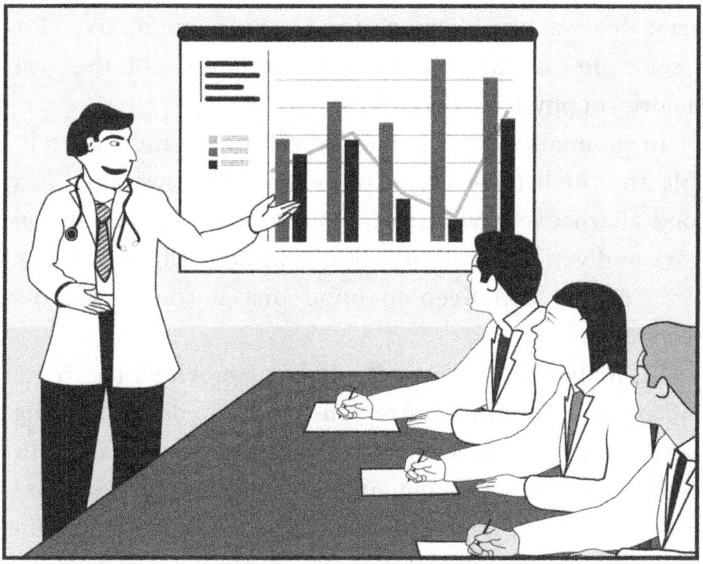

The path to becoming a physician executive is a step-by-step process. It begins by joining (unpaid) committees so that leaders get to know you. After several years of climbing the ladder, the administration department may buy some of your time at a comparable rate to what you are currently getting paid. In other words, it is only an *additional* compensation if you continue your clinical work and extend your after-hours work. Thus, you will continue to get similar pay but do less clinical work.

However, some institutions have a preset salary for administrative positions that tends to be higher than the average clinical rate. Many physicians like this idea and transition slowly to more admin as they decrease their clinical responsibilities. Keep in mind that, typically, the work is more hours than the time paid, and many will work both before *and* after hours. Some institutions do offer a 1–2% increase in salary every year, which is appealing in the long term. However, the big money and bonuses are reserved for a select few at the top of the institution, not the vast majority of physician executives.

In summary, I believe that clinical work is the most reliable and predictable source of income. Administration is a good alternative if you really want to cut back on clinical work and you enjoy administrative work. (Believe it or not, some people do.) Keep in mind that it comes with its headaches.

In my book, *No Work After Hours*, I provide tips, tricks, and philosophy to optimize your clinical work. Mastering the art of clinical efficiency can significantly increase your clinical revenue while remaining manageable. If you want to shift to admin work eventually, first maximize your clinical revenue so that the admin rate will also be very good.

7

BILLING FOR CLINICAL ENCOUNTERS

Don't compete on price. Compete on value.

— JEFFREY GIOTMER

Clinical encounters are the core of practice for many clinicians, and the rules for billing in outpatient settings are the same as for inpatient settings. These rules change and evolve, and I will do my best to keep updating this book to keep it current. The information here is current as of August 2024.

Historical Perspective

The old billing model focused excessively on the components of the chief complaint (cc), history of present illness (HPI), review of systems (ROS), past medical history (PMH), family history (FH), social history (SH), physical exam (PE), and medical decision-making (MDM) in the assessment and plan (A&P). For each billing level, you had to count the components in each category and ensure you didn't miss any. For instance, if you were seeing a new patient and planning to charge a moderate-complexity code based on the old 1995 guidelines, the requirements from the history and physical exam aspects were: ≥4 HPI elements, ≥10 ROS elements, three history areas (PMH, FH, and SH), and ≥ eight systems in PE. This was in addition to the MDM requirements, making it a real nightmare.

It was a daunting job to memorize and double-check all the requirements, and as you can imagine, the clinical notes were unnecessarily long. Under President Trump's administration, the requirements for clinical notes were significantly consolidated and focused only on the MDM in the 2021 Centers for Medicare and Medicaid Services (CMS) guidelines, which makes much more sense. In the old system, MDM was the core, but it was diluted with all the extensive requirements in the clinical note areas. Several coders reminded me that even if all the note's areas met the high-complexity charge in the old system, if the MDM was moderate complexity, then it should be coded as moderate complexity(!)

In this section, I won't focus on all the details of the current guidelines for billing and coding but rather on the crucial points that I find most useful. Your coder can give you a good briefing on the current guidelines and provide a cheat sheet; my aim is just to give you insider tips on maximizing your revenue.

Practical Applications for wRVU

For outpatient new visits, the CPT® charges (wRVU) for low, moderate, and high complexity are 99203 (1.6 wRVU), 99204 (2.6 wRVU), and 99205 (3.5 wRVU), respectively. Outpatient established visits are 99213 (1.3 wRVU), 99214 (1.92 wRVU), and 99215 (2.8 wRVU), respectively.

Did you notice that an established high-complexity outpatient visit earns more than a new moderate-complexity one? Did you notice that two established moderate-complexity visits will earn 3.84 wRVU while a moderate-complexity new visit is only 2.6 wRVU, a 47.7% more income? This is crucial to understand if your new patient visit slots are double the time of established visits. I believe this is a way that the Centers for Medicare and Medicaid Services (CMS) rewards the older, more experienced clinicians who have established practices with more established patients and fewer new patients. So, consider revisiting your template if you focus on seeing more new patients, especially if you assume they bring more revenue. On the other hand, if you can see the new patients in the same time slots as the established ones, you are on the right track.

For new inpatient patients, the CPT® charges for low, moderate, and high complexity are 99221 (1.63 wRVU), 99222 (2.6 wRVU), and 99223 (3.5 wRVU), respectively. For the follow-up inpatient patients, they are 99231 (0.76), 99232 (1.59 wRVU), and 99233 (2.4 wRVU), respectively. Notice that the wRVU values for the inpatient encounters are *less* than the outpatient; if your practice relies heavily on the inpatient service, do your math and weigh the pros and cons. For me, the inpatient consultation service is always a financial loss compared to the outpatient service, unless you have a high volume of new daily consults.

However, inpatient work does have several advantages I enjoy. I work closely with the fellows and residents, for example, which I love. It is a change in routine and keeps my skills up to date in inpatient service management. So, the package is acceptable to me, and I'm happy to do a few weeks per year.

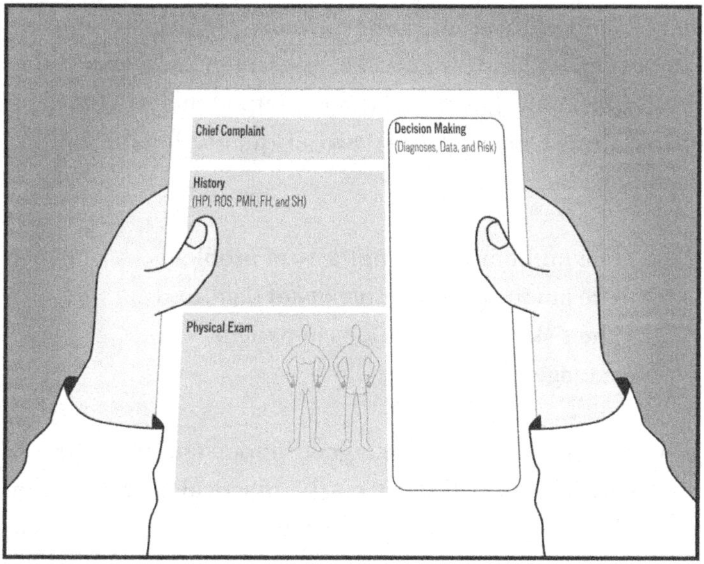

Chief Complaint

The chief complaint is the first line in any clinical note and represents why a patient is being seen in an outpatient clinical encounter. As silly as it sounds, it is a must in the old and current coding systems. You do not want to forget to write it. Keep in mind that auditors are sticklers for the rules and regulations. If there is no chief complaint, the note can be disqualified from being billable, and this can translate into you paying back money, sometimes a lot. If it isn't already, develop the habit of writing the chief complaint at the beginning of every note until it is automatic.

Medical Decision Making

Medical decision-making (MDM) is at the core of both charges and clinical encounters. Many physicians jump to this section to understand the assessment and make the plan right away. There are three components to consider, and you must meet at least two to qualify for the billing level. These are:

1. The number and complexity of problems,
2. The amount and complexity of data, and
3. The risk of complications in patient management.

I trust you already have a good understanding of these requirements, so I will focus on the practical aspects of the updated 2021 CMS billing and coding guidelines. If you need to become more familiar with them, please have a detailed session with your coder to understand the ins and outs. Billing is your business, and you should master it.

The MDM section is the core of our clinical practice and, of course, the patient's best interest should always be our main guide. If only a single problem allows me to bill for high complexity, but other pressing issues need to be addressed in the same visit, I will take care of them as well. We should always strive for a balanced approach to optimize both patient care and revenue while maintaining a reasonable workflow to reduce the risk of burnout.

Some software programs will review clinical notes and determine the level of coding accordingly. I wholeheartedly dislike these programs because, as we have discussed, when it comes to billing and coding, you need to find opportunities to maximize your revenue rather than play it safe. For example, I can bill a patient presentation as high-complexity that my colleague will bill as low complexity, and the auditor will find that both charges are correct. This depends on the phrasing that you write in the note to justify the billing level, which requires you to have in-depth knowledge of what to look for and how to write the notes.

Every medical and surgical specialty is unique, and I recommend digesting the guidelines well and tailoring them to your practice.

Number and Complexity of Problems

In medical billing, the complexity level of the care provided is determined by the status of the diagnoses rather than just the number of diagnoses. A single chronic problem, for instance, can justify billing for low, moderate, or high complexity. As previously mentioned, the number and complexity of problems is one of the three key categories in MDM. To meet the billing criteria, you need to fulfill two out of the three categories at the required level of complexity.

For a moderate-complexity charge, one chronic problem that is 'uncontrolled' or 'not at goal' is sufficient. For instance, a patient with type 2 diabetes and an A1c level of 7.1% is considered 'not at goal' if the target is <7%. Under 'diagnosis', I would list this as "Chronic, not at goal" or "Chronic, uncontrolled."

An alternative for billing a moderate-complexity charge is having two well-controlled chronic problems. For instance, a patient with well-controlled hypothyroidism and well-controlled dyslipidemia would meet this criterion. In such cases, I would document each condition with the notation: "Chronic, well controlled." My goal is to make the auditor's life easier and help them find the exact words as per the CMS guidelines.

A single problem with severe exacerbation, progression or side effects of treatment will qualify as a high-complexity charge. For example, a patient with heart failure and a significant acute kidney injury due to an increased dose of a diuretic; a patient with diabetes who is having severe hypoglycemic episodes due to insulin therapy; or a patient with osteoporosis who has had a hip fracture. These are all considered severe exacerbations. In such cases, my first line after the diagnosis line would be something like: "Notable severe exacerbation with current evidence of severe hypoglycemic episodes, a severe side effect of insulin therapy."

Amount and Complexity of Data

There are three broad categories under this section:

1. **Orders:** This includes ordering labs, imaging studies, or procedures.
2. **Independent Review of a Test:** This refers to the independent interpretation of a test performed by another physician.
3. **Discussion with Colleagues:** This involves consultation or discussion with other healthcare professionals regarding the patient's care.

To qualify for moderate complexity, you need to include one of these categories in your notes; for high complexity, you need to include two. This may sound like a lot of work, but believe me, it is far less than the amount of studying you did to become a physician. And, of course, it is well worth it as the improvement in your justified coding intensity can significantly increase your revenue.

For category 1 (orders), you need three elements to qualify for moderate complexity. For example, ordering tests for TSH, free T4, and total T3 — each with its own CPT® code — would qualify as three separate orders. If this patient is new, and you review these three lab tests and mention them in the notes, you will also have met the requirement. However, you can't order them for one visit, review them on the subsequent visit, and rely on them in *both* instances, i.e. you can't 'double-dip'. There are other limitations based on how tests are coded. For example, a renal panel has a single CPT® code, so the sodium, potassium, and creatinine levels given in a panel count as a single order.

Category 1 also includes reviewing prior external notes from each unique source and assessments requiring an independent historian. For instance, a primary care physician (PCP) reviewing notes for the same patient from a cardiologist, nephrologist, and endocrinologist — three unique sources — meets the moderate-complexity requirement, even if all are within the same EHR system. Just be sure to document this clearly, for example, state for each source: "I have personally reviewed the notes of **** and noted ****" under the corresponding problem. You don't need to include everything; just document three elements, which can be mixed and matched as needed.

Category 2 includes the independent review of the details of test results performed by another colleague, for example, an ultrasound, CT, MRI, or EKG done elsewhere. To qualify, you must not be charging for this review.

As part of my thyroid practice, I regularly perform and order thyroid ultrasound exams. Let's say I have a new patient being evaluated for thyrotoxicosis who had labs (TSH, free T4, and total T3) and a thyroid ultrasound completed by their PCP before our visit. My review of these labs, documented in my notes, meets the moderate-complexity requirement. I will also review the images of relevant studies, such as thyroid ultrasounds, and will include screenshots in my notes with a statement like: "I personally reviewed the images of the thyroid ultrasound from 1/2024, noting pseudo-nodules and hypervascularity. No current indication for follow-up exams unless new issues arise." This documents my assessment of the images.

Thus, reviewing the three lab results and providing an independent interpretation constitutes a high-complexity component of Category 2. For similar patients, I also often perform a spectral Doppler ultrasound during the initial visit to assess peak systolic velocities of various thyroid arteries. This constitutes an additional charge, and it is reported separately.

Discussing a patient's case with another provider, including through EHR-based messages, qualifies as additional data complexity and is sufficient on its own to meet the moderate-complexity requirement. Again, you need to document this clearly, for example, with a statement in the notes such as: "I have personally discussed ****'s case with Dr. **** and agreed upon ****."

We follow many steps to provide good patient care. It's essential to practice clear and accurate note-taking to document each step properly so we qualify for the correct complexity level. Let's go through an example. Below is a section of the MDM for a new patient with thyrotoxicosis, for which I billed high complexity (CPT® 99205) and a spectral Doppler ultrasound (CPT® 93880):

Graves Disease E05.0:

- *Notable evidence of severe exacerbation with a recent hospital admission for atrial fibrillation, a severe disease-related progression.*
- *Symptoms started around 11/2023, including palpitations, tremors, heat intolerance, and unintentional weight loss of 30 Ibs.*
- *Noted labs 2/2024 TSH < 0.01, FT4 4.9, and total T3 495.*
- *I have personally reviewed the images of the thyroid ultrasound in 2/2024. There were no nodules, but hypervascularity and thyromegaly were noted.*
- *I have personally performed a separately reported spectral Doppler ultrasound today, PSV up to 70 cm/sec, consistent with Graves' disease."*

In this example, the first bullet point demonstrates the high complexity of the single problem, which qualifies the case for a high-complexity charge. The third and fourth bullet points document the high complexity of the data reviewed. As these meet two out of the three billing categories, this patient encounter will qualify for a high-complexity charge, whether this is a new or established patient. From a clinical standpoint, I documented the confirmed diagnosis in the notes based on my assessment, including the initial symptoms and my findings from the ultrasound I performed. These are important pieces of the clinical assessment and plan.

(For more on how to write efficient and comprehensive notes, see my book, *No Work After Hours*.)

Risk of Complication of Patient Management

The third and last major aspect of MDM is the risk of complications. In a nutshell, there are a few things you need to be familiar with.

Firstly, managing a medication, including whether to continue to hold or not to start it, qualifies for moderate complexity. For example, a patient with well-controlled osteoporosis who is currently on a drug holiday from Fosamax, for whom I order three lab tests to be done before the next consultation in one year's time, will qualify for moderate complexity. The charge is based on the amount of data, three labs, the risk of complications, and prescription drug management. Note that discussing major surgery with identified risks qualifies for high complexity, whereas discussing major surgery without identified risks qualifies for moderate-complexity.

For high-complexity charges, several factors should be considered. First, consider medications that require intensive monitoring for toxicity. The American Medical Association (AMA) provides examples like monitoring electrolytes in a patient on a diuretic — a common scenario. Note that monitoring must focus on toxicity rather than efficacy, be based on labs or imaging studies rather than history or physical exams and occur at least every three months; annual labs are insufficient. Examples include monitoring coagulation factors in patients on warfarin; BMP levels after starting losartan; spironolactone, or empagliflozin, or glucose levels in patients on insulin experiencing severe hypoglycemia. Ensure your documentation includes a clear statement describing the monitoring. For example: "The patient requires intensive monitoring of serum potassium and kidney function due to the risk of spironolactone-induced acute kidney injury and hyperkalemia. Check BMP before the follow-up in 3 months."

Other topics of discussion qualify for high complexity, such as the decision to not resuscitate or de-escalate care, a common discussion in some specialties. Another common example in some specialties is discussing an elective major surgical intervention with identified patient or procedure-related risks. For example, discussing subtotal parathyroidectomy in a patient with end-stage kidney disease and hypercalcemia due to tertiary hyperparathyroidism. This surgery is associated with risk of severe hypocalcemia due to 'hungry bone syndrome', and qualifies for high complexity, e.g.: "Discussed the benefits and hazards of subtotal parathyroidectomy today, an elective major surgery. The patient is at risk of severe hypocalcemia, a surgery-related risk."

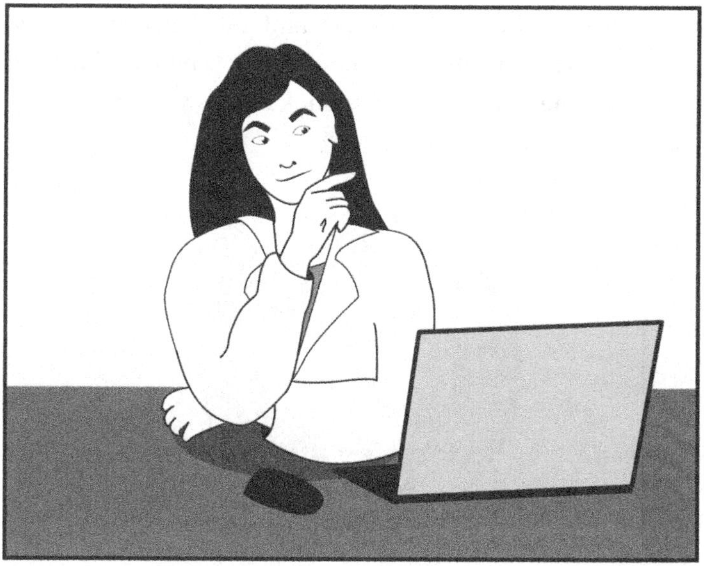

In Summary

The key point is that you need two out of the three elements in the MDM section to support high-complexity billing. This doesn't require extensive notes; a few lines under each problem will do. Patient care, of course, is of utmost importance and will always come first, but after this, it's important to focus on justifying proper billing for your work while being efficient with your time and effort. Essentially, this means writing a small range of phrases that satisfy the auditor who reviews your notes. In their random audits, your coder will provide valuable feedback. Ensure you take it seriously and modify your note-writing accordingly.

We are busy, and developing more detailed notes to defend your billing level might seem like an additional burden. Initially, it will be. But have faith that it will soon become automatic and eventually you won't need to refer to the billing and coding cheat sheet, and it will take only a few seconds to know what you need to write. The fact that you have taken the time to read this book means you are already in great shape, so keep it up.

8

CODERS AND AUDITORS

Quality is more important than quantity. One home run is much better than two doubles.

— STEVE JOBS

Remember when you first learned to drive? It took time and practice to understand the rules and what to do — and what not to do. Now, driving is second nature, and you automatically follow the rules. Occasionally, you might break a rule without being noticed. But sometimes you might find flashing lights behind you and get a warning or a ticket, and it may be expensive or cause you a headache in other ways.

Optimizing billing and coding is similar. It requires training to be an independent physician and accurately bill for your patients. Unfortunately, medical training focuses only on patient care and good medical practice, and the specifics of billing and coding are not taught. However, when you're audited, they don't focus on how great a caregiver you are, they focus on how accurate you are in following the well-defined coding practices. Mastering these practices is essential for running your business effectively.

How Do Payers Think?

Let's try a fun exercise. Close your eyes and imagine you're in a suit, sitting in a fancy meeting room. You are the CEO of a prominent private insurance company or a senior executive at a government healthcare payor. You're reviewing numerous financial reports and discussing billions of dollars. As you skim through graphs of trends and projections, what questions would you ask? What would be in the company's best interest? How would you leverage your position? What battles would you choose to fight? What are the easiest ways to save the organization money?

The job of leadership in any payor organization is to find ways to save money. Like any for-profit business, its job is to maximize net revenue, and it can generally only do this by increasing premiums and cutting back on expenses. Although government payers are not-for-profit, reducing healthcare-related expenses allows those funds to be allocated to other areas, which is beneficial. They still want to be fair and provide high-quality service, so they develop guidelines drafted by reputable clinicians. Additionally, they implement controls, such as prior authorizations, to prevent automatic payments for unnecessary or excessively expensive services.

As clinicians, we are alert to how insurers look at our charges. Frankly speaking, we are one of the less expensive components of healthcare expenses. In an interesting article in *Missouri Medicine*, Timothy B. Norbeck notes that physicians account for only about 10% of health care expenses. Rising expenses, he argues, are primarily driven by administrative costs, hospitals, pharmaceuticals, and severe comorbidities, rather than by physicians.

Yet physicians simultaneously face both progressive cuts in revenue and rising inflation. Payers will continue to push to lower costs and will fight for every penny, and the stronger side will win. If you work for a large institution, it will have significant leverage in negotiating reimbursement rates. They are powerful and will determine your pay based on the wRVU rate they set and adjust it according to their business needs. On the other hand, if you have a small private practice, you will have weak negotiating power, and you may have to agree to lower fees and higher patient volume.

Auditors

Another way a healthcare payor saves money is by hiring auditors to identify and recover funds from overpayments or billing errors. They have different ranks, each with a different mission. Here is a list from the Centers for Medicare and Medicaid Services (CMS), and you can read more about them here.

- **Medicare Administrative Contractors (MACs):** Process Medicare claims, enroll healthcare providers, and educate providers on Medicare billing requirements.
- **Recovery Audit Contractors (RACs):** These are headhunters. They are paid on a contingency fee basis, and they audit retrospectively.
- **Comprehensive Error Rate Testing contractors (CERTs):** Auditor of the auditors who ensure that MACs and RACs are doing their job correctly.

- **Zone Program Integrity Contractors (ZPICs):** Investigate fraud and abuse.

Auditors review random samples of clinical notes and compare their components against the well-defined CMS guidelines for billing and coding. Based on this assessment, they decide whether charges are accurate or overcharged.

There are several challenging aspects to audits. Firstly, auditors can be biased. They have a conflict of interest because their bonuses increase with the amount of money they recover. They typically review a small random sample of records and extrapolate their findings. For example, if an auditor reviews 30 notes and finds that 10 were overcharged by $50 each, they might assume that one-third of all notes billed by that physician are similarly overcharged. If that physician submitted 1,200 notes to the payor over the past five years, this could result in an extrapolated overcharge of $20,000, which the physician is requested to pay back. Other scenarios might involve even larger 'overcharges'.

Another challenge is that auditors are not physicians, and although they may have a bachelor's or a master's degree, they usually do not have a medical background. For one thing, it would be too expensive to employ physicians as auditors. Consequently, auditors may not understand complex medical abbreviations or terminology. When writing your notes, keep them simple, concise, and aligned with CMS guidelines. This ensures clarity and accuracy, which is why my dot phrases frequently include the exact wording used by CMS.

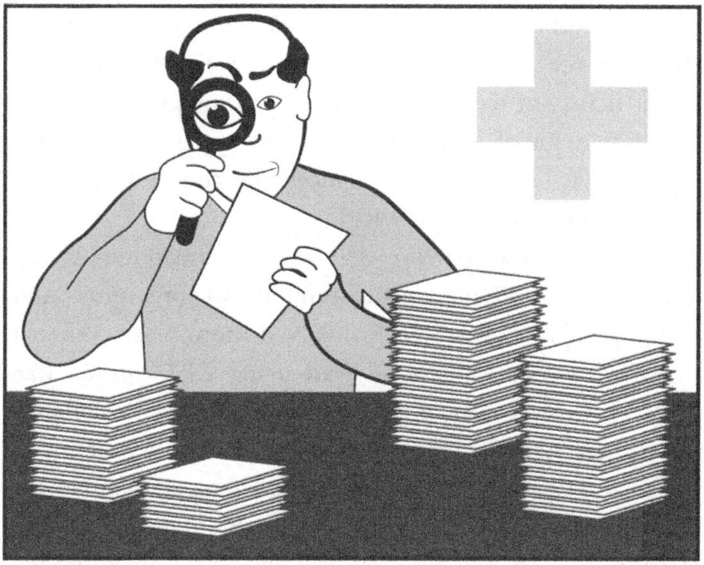

Your Coder

Your coder is extremely valuable. They understand CMS guidelines, have a background similar to auditors, and can provide valuable advice and guidance. I have contacted my coders many times, for example, to check the accuracy of my dot phrases for certain billing requirements. I have also benefited from their internal audits.

Coders can suggest new codes to use that you were previously unaware of. You don't know what you don't know. For example, I started using my ultrasound machine to measure the thyroidal artery pressure in patients with thyrotoxicosis. The general practice among endocrinologists is to do formal thyroid ultrasound exams, CPT® 76536, 0.56 wRVU. If there are no thyroid nodules and the exam is straightforward, I will capture 13 images as well as another 5 for the measurements. It takes 15 to 25 minutes to capture the images, transfer them to the EHR, and write the report. This is quite a long time, partly as we don't have the infrastructure or technicians that the radiology department has. It is a lot of work and has a minimal wRVU value compared to, for example, a moderate-complexity established patient earning 1.92 wRVU.

Initially, I was performing formal ultrasounds along with spectral Doppler measurements of pressures, and charging CPT® 76536, which involved more work. When I consulted my coder, she advised using CPT® 93880 (0.8 wRVU) if I measured the spectral Doppler pressures bilaterally without needing additional images of the thyroid gland. She also assisted with the phrasing of my notes. Now, I capture only four images, obtain valuable data for clinical decision-making, and increase my revenue. This approach has become standard practice in my clinic for assessing new consults for thyrotoxicosis.

Your coder can also offer other suggestions. For example, I learned I can incorporate procedure notes into my E/M notes. This means that, from a billing and coding perspective, it's acceptable to incorporate the interpretation of continuous glucose monitors, thyroid ultrasounds, spectral Doppler ultrasounds, thyroid biopsies, or thyroid ablation procedures into your regular consult or progress notes. This has made my life easier and more streamlined. There are likely similar tips for your specialty and practice.

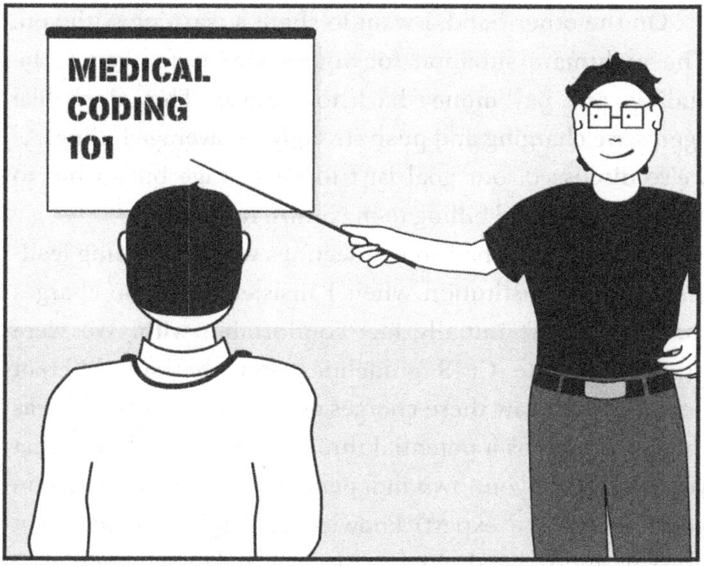

Life in billing and coding is dynamic and continuously changing. Like medicine, you need to keep up to date. Coders are a big help here and can, for example, update you on new codes and charges specific to your specialty. Consider marking your calendar annually around early December to get updates for the following year. CMS usually releases the physician fee schedule updates in early November, and they can also help update you on that.

My advice is, if you are in doubt, reach out and ask your coder. It's a win-win situation: you might learn something new, while they will feel appreciated and valued. Don't underestimate this; we physicians have a high value in the eyes of those working around us. Imagine that the CEO is asking for your expertise and valuing it, how would you feel? Building a positive rapport can encourage them to delve deeper and provide you with even more valuable insights.

On the other hand, I want to share a warning with you. The nightmare situation for your coder is for you to be audited and pay money back to a payer. They don't like aggressive charging and push strongly for average billing. As we've discussed, our goal isn't to be average billers but to master coding and billing to maximize revenue.

On this note, I had some meetings with the coding leadership at my institution when I insisted on some charges that they didn't initially feel comfortable with. We were using the same CMS guidelines, but we had different perspectives. I saw these charges as an opportunity whereas they saw them as a potential threat. The bottom line is that you need to do your own independent assessment based on your (soon-to-be expert) knowledge. Don't overshoot, but don't be intimidated either; aim for a balanced confidence grounded in a solid foundation of knowledge.

9

IN CONCLUSION

I'm a great believer in luck, and I find the harder I work, the more I have of it.

— THOMAS JEFFERSON

As much as I enjoy caring for patients, and it is very fulfilling, I find the billing and coding an exciting game. Like any game — sports, board, or video games — there is a learning curve. And when you finish one level, you move on to the next. The same applies to learning billing, coding, and various practice tweaks to improve your efficiency, effectiveness, and productivity. And the good thing is that there is no 'finish line', it is a path of continuous improvement and progressive growth.

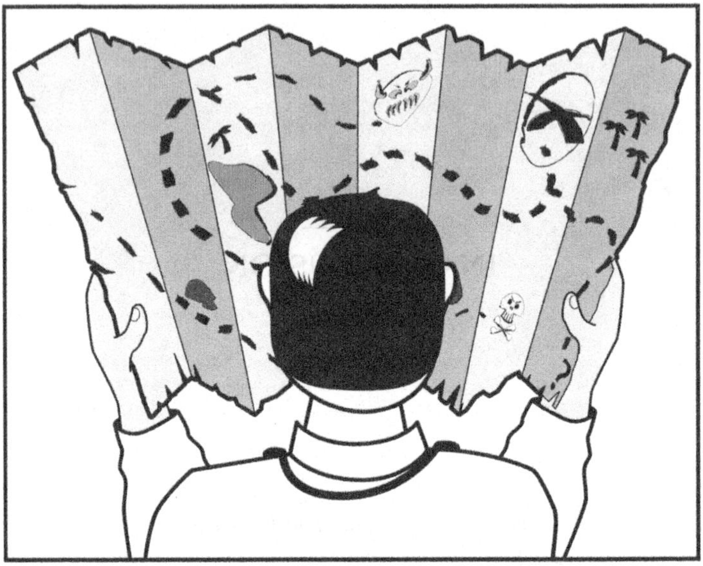

Continuous Education

As physicians, we need continuous medical education (CME) to keep our knowledge current. We attend conferences, listen to webinars, and read articles. We should treat billing, coding, and practice management in the same way. Grasp every opportunity to learn and improve your knowledge. Unfortunately, there is not much information out there, but use what you have and keep searching.

If you want to go further than a book can take you, I built a course for exactly that. Physician Revenue & Efficiency Mastery is the full version of what you have just read: level-by-level billing walk-throughs on real encounter types, medical decision-making scenarios with the reasoning made explicit, how auditors actually think and how to defend your billing, the compensation math you need before you sign a contract — and, on the efficiency side, the systems that let you finish clinic work inside clinic hours.

The course is CME-accredited through a jointly accredited provider, so your institution's CME allowance will in most cases cover the cost. Full accreditation and credit details are on the course page. Ask your administrator. Physicians are frequently surprised to learn they have unspent funds sitting there.

You can see it and take the free training at the link below.

go.mdefficacy.com/mastery

Physician Revenue & Efficiency Mastery

Beyond that: my website, vlog, blog, and social media pages are free. There are also many online groups for various specialties and practice types, and the discussions there are very useful. I believe that sharing experience among colleagues is priceless. I usually start by sharing some information about my practice, and magically, others feel safe sharing theirs as well. Bouncing ideas and learning from other models is a great way to improve.

Share the Benefit

If you learned some tips and enjoyed this book, please recommend it to a colleague. Spreading knowledge goes a long way. Also, I would appreciate it if you could take a minute to leave a review on Amazon.com and Goodreads.-com, which will help many others benefit from your experience.

If you have thoughts, feedback, questions, or concerns, please don't hesitate to email me at the email below.

info@MDEfficacy.com

MD EFFICACY

EFFECTIVENESS EFFICIENCY ®

YOUR NEXT STEP

A book can give you the map. It cannot walk the route with you. If the chapters on medical decision making, coding, and compensation models opened up questions rather than closing them, that is the correct reaction. This material rewards depth, and depth is difficult to deliver in print.

That is why I built Physician Revenue & Efficiency Mastery. It teaches this material the way I wish someone had taught me during fellowship:

- Level-by-level billing walk-throughs on real encounter types
- Medical decision-making scenarios with the reasoning made explicit
- How auditors think, and how to defend your billing when they come
- The hands-on revenue tracking tools you need to lead your practice with power
- The efficiency systems I use to run the busiest clinic in my division and still leave when clinic ends

Billing correctly does not help you if you are still charting at ten at night. Revenue and efficiency are the same problem viewed from two sides, which is why I teach them together.

The course is CME-accredited through a jointly accredited provider, so your institution's CME allowance will in most cases cover the cost. Full accreditation and credit details are on the course page. Ask your administrator. Physicians are frequently surprised to learn they have unspent funds sitting there.

Start with the free training at the link below, and leave your email. I'll send you my revenue tracking sheet, a tutorial on using it, and my EHR keyboard shortcuts, at no cost and with no obligation.

go.mdefficacy.com/mastery

Physician Revenue & Efficiency Mastery

Questions before you decide? Email me directly at the email below. I read and answer them myself.

info@MDEfficacy.com

ACKNOWLEDGMENTS

This book is the result of cumulative information collection from various sources.

I would like to first thank the American Association of Clinical Endocrinology (AACE) for providing billing and coding courses, and Rush University Medical Center for its year-long career guidance series. Both have been invaluable guides on my journey.

Many physicians, clinicians, educators, executive leaders, and scientists have generously shared their valuable experiences with me. I would like to thank the physicians listed below, who have greatly contributed to my understanding of productivity over the years and during the writing of this book. They are listed in alphabetical order by last name, followed by their specialty and area of expertise.

- Dr. Melissa Cavaghan: Endocrinologist, academic and service line leader
- Dr. Sherif Dawood: Ophthalmologist, academic and private practice
- Dr. Michael Econs: Endocrinologist, academic chairman, and physician-scientist
- Dr. Michael Hanna: Pain management specialist, academic and private practice
- Dr. Olena Klindukhova: Endocrinologist, academic and private practice

- Dr. Jyothi Mamidi Juarez: Endocrinologist, private practice
- Dr. Noah Parker: ENT surgeon, academic and private practice
- Dr. Shant Parseghian: Endocrinologist, academic and private practice
- Dr. Zeb Saeed: Academic Endocrinologist and physician educator
- Dr. Viral Shah: Academic Endocrinologist and scientist
- Dr. Rocky Singh: Chief Medical Officer
- Dr. Chad Zarse: Academic Nephrologist

I would also like to thank Jennifer Poyter, the physician coding expert at IU Health, where I practice, for all the support and guidance, and IU Health's endocrinology practice administrator, Tonya Somers, for her thoughtful input.

The Endocrine Society and AACE continue to provide insights, guidance, and support, for which I am grateful. I also appreciate Mary Todd's professional help in editing the manuscript and Mike Trent's illustrations for the book cover and interior illustrations.

ABOUT THE AUTHOR

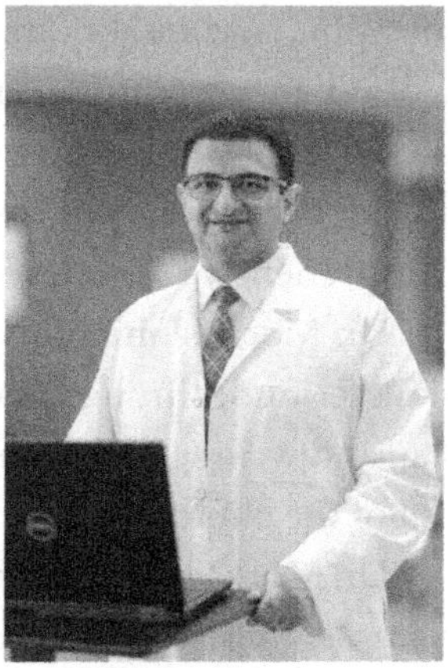

Dr. Michael Morkos, Associate Professor of Clinical Medicine at Indiana University School of Medicine, specializes in endocrinology and metabolism. Passionate about the business of medicine, he completed extensive coursework in business during his master's degree in health informatics and received formal coding education. He is dedicated to supporting physicians by highlighting and addressing the significant gaps in their understanding of the business aspects of medical practice.

After earning his medical degree from Alexandria University in Egypt, he completed his internal medicine residency at John H. Stroger Jr. Hospital of Cook County and his endocrinology fellowship at Rush University Medical Center. He holds master's degrees in clinical research and healthcare informatics and is board-certified in internal medicine, endocrinology, and clinical informatics.

Dr. Morkos is the founder of MD Efficacy and is publishing a series of books to help physicians improve clinic efficiency and productivity while maintaining excellent patient outcomes. He specializes in thyroid disorders and co-directs Indiana's only multidisciplinary thyroid and parathyroid center. As a pioneer in thyroid radiofrequency ablation and a rare user of spectral Doppler ultrasound for thyrotoxicosis, he integrates clinical excellence with cutting-edge technology.

His expertise extends to statistical analysis, EHR optimization, and quality improvement, enhanced by his background in accounting and business. A dedicated mentor, public speaker, and church leader, he is committed to advancing physicians' efficacy and patient care through comprehensive skill development.

Dr. Morkos' mission is to continue to develop his broad skill set and, through mentorship, coaching, public speaking, and writing, enhance the lives of physicians both in and out of the clinic.

Dr. Morkos teaches this material in depth through *Physician Revenue & Efficiency Mastery*, MD Efficacy's CME-accredited course for physicians, available with free training and a free revenue-tracking sheet at the link below.

go.mdefficacy.com/mastery

Physician Revenue & Efficiency Mastery

facebook.com/MDEfficacy

x.com/MDEfficacy

linkedin.com/company/mdefficacy

youtube.com/@MDEfficacy

ALSO BY MICHAEL MORKOS, MD

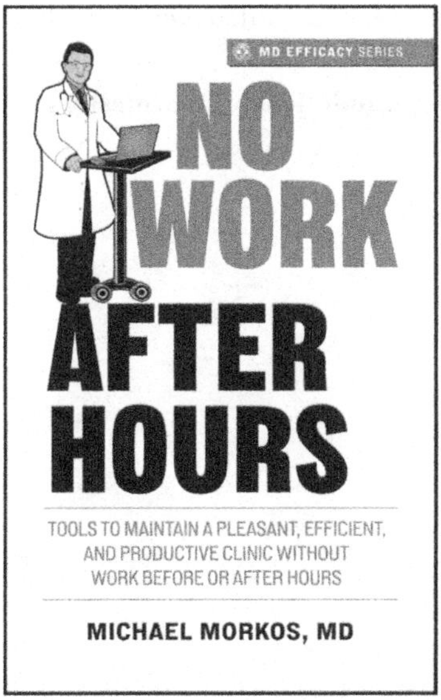

No Work After Hours: Tools to Maintain a Pleasant, Efficient, and Productive Clinic Without Work Before or After Hours — Book 1 in the MD Efficacy series.

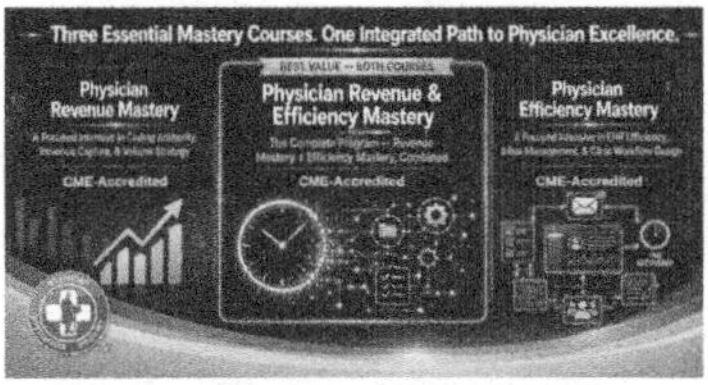

The MD Efficacy course series — revenue, efficiency, or both.

Physician Revenue Mastery: a focused intensive in coding authority, revenue capture, and volume strategy.

Physician Efficiency Mastery: a focused intensive in EHR efficiency, inbox management, and clinic workflow design.

Physician Revenue & Efficiency Mastery: the complete program, both courses combined.

All three are CME-accredited. Details at the link below.

go.mdefficacy.com/mastery

Made in the USA
Monee, IL
13 September 2026

62976619R00079